A Manual of Systematic Eyelid Surgery

Commissioning Editor: Paul Fam
Project Development Manager: Tim Kimber
Project Manager: Kathryn Mason
Design Manager: Jayne Jones
Illustration Manager: Mick Ruddy
Illustrator: Paul Richardson
Marketing Managers: Gaynor Jones (UK)/Lisa Damico (USA)

A Manual of Systematic Eyelid Surgery

THIRD EDITION

J.R.O. Collin MA MB BChir FRCS FRCOpth DO
Consultant Surgeon,
Moorfields Eye Hospital and Institute of Ophthalmology,
University of London;

Honorary Consultant Ophthalmic Surgeon,
The Hospitals for Sick Children,
Great Ormond Street, London, UK

BUTTERWORTH
HEINEMANN

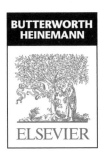

ELSEVIER

**BUTTERWORTH
HEINEMANN**
ELSEVIER

ISBN 0-7506-4550-4

British Library Cataloguing in Publication Data
A catalogue record for this book is available from the British Library

Library of Congress Cataloging in Publication Data
A catalog record for this book is available from the Library of Congress

Notice
Medical knowledge is constantly changing. Standard safety precautions must be followed, but as new research and clinical experience broaden our knowledge, changes in treatment and drug therapy may become necessary or appropriate. Readers are advised to check the most current product information provided by the manufacturer of each drug to be administered to verify the recommended dose, the method and duration of administration, and contraindications. It is the responsibility of the practitioner, relying on experience and knowledge of the patient, to determine dosages and the best treatment for each individual patient. Neither the Publisher nor the author assume any liability for any injury and/or damage to persons or property arising from this publication.

The Publisher

Printed in the United Kingdom
Last digit is the print number: 9 8 7 6 5 4 3 2 1

Contents

Preface

This Manual is written for all surgeons and ophthalmologists who operate on eyelids. Its purpose is to promote a systematic approach to eyelid and lacrimal surgery and to simplify the choice of operation. Flow charts are used, which allow the reader to see at a glance which is the most appropriate procedure for any given set of circumstances. Each operation is described under the headings of 'Principle', 'Indications', 'Method' and 'Complications'. A large number of simple diagrams have been included to make the text as clear as possible. Alternative operations are largely omitted in the interests of clarity and brevity. No attempt is made to be encyclopaedic and if the reader wants to explore any aspect in greater detail, a list of books for suggested further reading is included at the end of the first chapter. This 'system' has been used successfully at Moorfields Eye Hospital for the last 25 years but the book also includes minor modifications which may make it more appropriate to other parts of the world with different operating conditions.

In this third edition complications have been added as a separate heading for each operation reflecting the recognised need to inform patients about these prior to surgery. The layout of the chapters has been changed. Simple basic procedures such as wound closure and taking different grafts have been collected in one place, Chapter 2, where they can easily be referenced. The chapter on ectropion has been rewritten. There are new chapters on important topics such as facial palsy and thyroid eye disease. The chapters on socket and cosmetic surgery have been considerably expanded and updated, reflecting the advances in these subjects. There are new flow charts and the old ones have been modified and expanded but the basic format of the book is the same. With the retirement of the original artist, Terry Tarrant, line diagrams have been replaced with shaded drawings which I hope will help identification and clarity without loss of simplicity and accuracy. With all these additions and modifications, the book is inevitably larger but the improvements should bring the book up to date and hopefully enhance its value as a simple basic practical guide to all who practice eyelid surgery.

London, 2006   J.R.O.C.

Dedicated to my family, Geraldine, Sophie and Olivia and to my trainees, colleagues and friends, without whose help, support and encouragement this book would never have been written.

Acknowledgements

This book would never have been written without the help, stimulation and example of all those who taught and influenced me, in particular, Crowell Beard from the University of California, San Francisco, Barrie Jones from Moorfields Eye Hospital and Jack Mustardé from Scotland. Sadly, since the last edition, Crowell Beard has died but his legacy lives on. With his typical modesty he would not allow me to give him the recognition he deserved and it was limited in previous editions to a dedication to 'C.B.' I can now freely acknowledge my debt to him and his enormous contribution to teaching ocular plastic surgery in the world. His various fellows have in their turn taught and influenced others but, as I have learnt, teaching is a circle and those who are being taught also contribute to the subject and to their teacher. I am certainly in

debted to my registrars, fellows and colleagues to whose influence many of the changes in this edition are due. The book has been extensively rewritten and much has been changed. The flow charts have been retained and the credit for their concept remains with Doug Coster from Adelaide, without whose encouragement and help the first edition would not have been written. Dick Welham kindly wrote the chapter on lacrimal surgery for the second edition and this has been altered very little. My thanks are also due to Sarah Sanders without whose tireless secretarial efforts this third edition would never have got to the publisher.

Surgical anatomy and general principles

1

This chapter emphasises some of the anatomical details and general considerations which are relevant to lid surgery. It is not intended to be a precise account of eyelid anatomy.

SKIN

Upper lid skin is thin and allows mobility of the eyelid. It stretches with age and there is usually excess available for a full-thickness skin graft. This takes well because there is no subcutaneous fat. The skin is thicker below the brow laterally and this makes an excellent graft for a lower eyelid defect. By contrast, there is often no vertical excess lower eyelid skin. The excision of skin lesions on the lower lid should be made as vertically as possible to avoid an ectropion. Incisions in the upper lid should preferably be made in the skin crease. When a graft or flap of thick skin is sutured to the thin eyelid skin, a small bite should be taken of the thick skin and a large bite of the thin skin to give the best result.

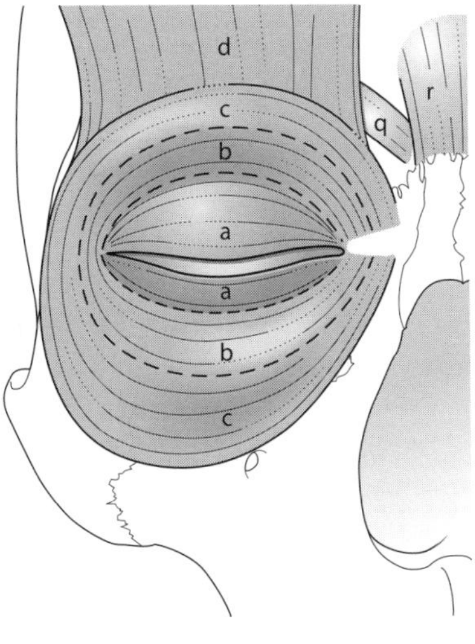

ORBICULARIS MUSCLE (Fig 1.1)

The orbital part of the orbicularis muscle (Fig 1.1c) surrounds the orbital rim and is responsible for forced eyelid closure. Skin creases are created at right angles to the line of contraction of any muscle. The action of the orbital part of the orbicularis muscle therefore forms creases or wrinkles beyond the lateral canthus (rhytides or 'crows feet'). These increase with age. The excessive action of the orbital orbicularis muscle can be reduced with botulinum toxin but excess toxin will cause lagophthalmos in the upper lid and a lower lid ectropion.

The palpebral part of the orbicularis muscle is artificially divided into a pretarsal muscle (Fig 1.1a), in front of the tarsal plate, and a preseptal muscle (Fig 1.1b), in front of the orbital septum in each lid. Each pretarsal muscle arises from the lateral canthal tendon and inserts by two heads. The superficial heads form the superficial part of the medial canthal tendon and the deep

Figure 1.1

heads insert onto the bone of the posterior lacrimal crest, forming the posterior limb of the medial canthal tendon. When the muscle contracts it closes the lid and pulls the lacrimal puncta medially into the lacus lacrimalis. Each preseptal muscle similarly inserts by a superficial and deep head. The superficial heads form the superficial part of the medial canthal tendon and the deep heads insert into the lacrimal fascia on the lateral side of the lacrimal sac. When the muscle contracts the lacrimal fascia is pulled laterally, creating a relative vacuum in the lacrimal sac at the same time as the pretarsal muscle pulls the puncta medially into the lacus lacrimalis. Tears enter the lacrimal sac. When the muscles relax the lacrimal fascia returns to normal and tears pass down the nasolacrimal duct.

Involutional changes affect the orbicularis muscle and its connective tissue and tendons. In involutional entropion, histopathological changes are present in the muscle itself. Connective tissue laxity allows the preseptal muscle to move upwards and the lid inverts. In involutional ectropion the preseptal muscle is relatively tethered to the lower border of the tarsus and the same involutional changes produce an eversion of the lid. Laxity of the medial and lateral canthal tendons may be due to involutional or paralytic changes.

The normal muscle is very efficient at closing the eyelids and it is extremely difficult to limit eyelid closure by the excision of orbicularis muscle, as has been tried for the treatment of blepharospasm. This means that the lid can be relatively freely 'debulked' during operations without prejudicing eyelid closure. The muscle is supplied by branches of the seventh nerve which tend to run vertically as they approach the lid margins. Vertical eyelid incisions therefore do not denervate the muscle. When it is cut, the muscle contracts and pulls the fragments of the eyelid apart. These eyelid fragments must be pulled together to overcome the contraction of the orbicularis muscle and laxity of the medial and lateral canthal tendons before deciding on a repair.

ORBITAL SEPTUM (Fig 1.2)

This is a tough sheet of fibrous tissue (Fig 1.2b') which is firmly attached to the orbital rim and more loosely attached to the lid retractors (Fig 1.2e). It divides the eyelids from the orbit. If the orbital rim is fractured the lid can be retracted by these attachments. The septum can be felt as a tight band under the orbicularis muscle when traction is exerted on it during an operation. This limitation of movement differentiates it from the fibrous tissue of the aponeurosis, which is mobile because of its attachment to the levator muscle. The septum must be cut to mobilise the lids fully in any lid reconstruction procedure or to expose the lid retractors, e.g. for a ptosis or lower lid retractor plication operation.

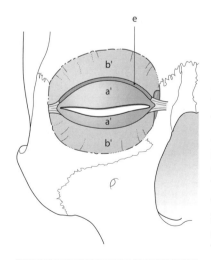

Figure 1.2

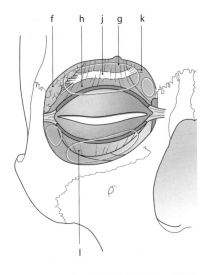

Figure 1.3

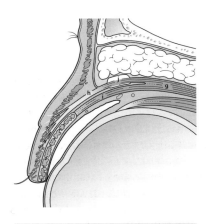

Figure 1.4

PREAPONEUROTIC FAT PAD (Fig 1.3)

This lies immediately behind the orbital septum (Fig 1.3, dotted lines). In the upper lid the fat is partially divided into a medial and central compartment. The lacrimal gland lies laterally (Fig 1.3f). It is important to remember this when excising fat from the upper lid for a blepharoplasty. In the lower lid the fat is partially divided into a larger central and smaller lateral fat pad. Blood vessels run through the fibrous septa in the fat pads. Traction on the fat pads should be avoided since it may lead to rupture of these septa and vessels deep in the orbit. This is a potential cause of blindness. The fat pads lie in front of the lid retractors. This relationship is invaluable in the identification of the aponeurosis and levator muscle in the upper lid, and of the retractors in the lower lid.

UPPER LID RETRACTORS (Fig 1.4)

The striated levator muscle (Figs 1.3g, 1.4g) arises from the lesser wing of the sphenoid and extends forwards for about 40 mm before it splits into the aponeurosis (Figs 1.3h, 1.4h) and the superior tarsal (Müller's) muscle (Fig 1.4i). It is supplied by the superior division of the third nerve by a branch which runs through the superior rectus muscle. Simple congenital ptosis is caused by a dysgenesis of the muscle, and the levator function is directly related to the extent of the dysgenetic changes in the muscle.

The aponeurosis (Figs 1.3h, 1.4h) is a dense sheet of collagen fibres which arises from the striated levator muscle and inserts between the orbicularis muscle bundles to form the skin crease. It spreads out medially and laterally under the superior suspensory (Whitnall's) ligament (Figs 1.3j, 1.4j) and inserts adjacent to the medial and lateral canthal tendons, forming the 'horns of the levator'. If the levator aponeurosis stretches or disinserts the skin crease rises which is a feature of ptosis caused by an aponeurotic weakness. The orbital septum blends with the aponeurosis superiorly. The preaponeurotic fat pad lies behind the orbital septum and above the aponeurosis. This acts as an invaluable aid in its identification during surgery.

The superior tarsal (Müller's) muscle (Fig 1.4i) extends as a thin strip of smooth muscle from the striated levator muscle to the upper border of the tarsal plate. The aponeurosis lies anterior to it and the conjunctiva posterior to it. The smooth muscle cells arise adjacent to the terminal striated muscle cells of the levator and insert into the tarsal plate via a 1 mm tendon. It is supplied by sympathetic nerves which are probably carried to it around blood vessels. Denervation causes the ptosis of Horner's syndrome.

The upper lid is lifted by the action of the levator muscle and the height is adjusted by the superior tarsal (Müller's) muscle. The levator complex is supported anteriorly by the superior suspensory

(Whitnall's) ligament (Figs 1.3j, 1.4j) which runs from the lacrimal gland capsule to the trochlea of the superior oblique muscle (Fig 1.3k). It has a thinner inferior part which encircles the levator muscle. The frontalis muscle (Fig 1.1d) contributes to elevation of the lid by lifting the brow. The superior tarsal (Müller's) muscle, the aponeurosis, the levator muscle, the frontalis muscle and the superior suspensory (Whitnall's) ligament can all be used to lift the eyelid, as will be discussed in the chapter on ptosis surgery.

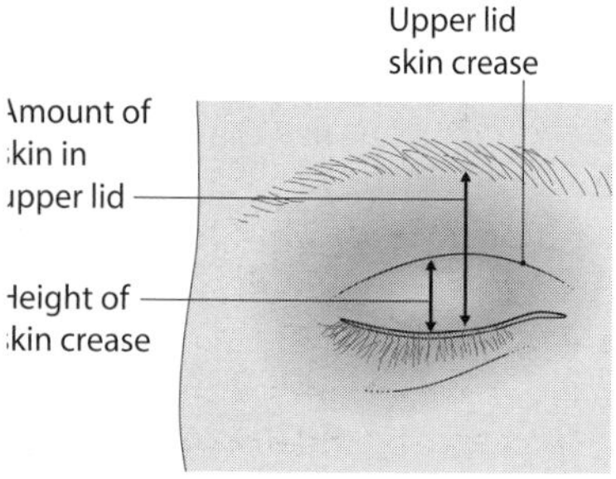

SKIN CREASE (Figs 1.4, 1.5, 1.6)

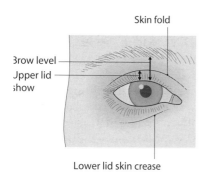

Upper lid skin crease

Amount of skin in upper lid

Height of skin crease

Figure 1.5

This is formed by the insertion of the levator aponeurosis into the orbicularis muscle bundles and postorbicularis fascia (Fig 1.4 h). It is measured by its height above the eyelid margin when it first becomes clinically apparent as the patient starts to look up from a position of down gaze (Fig 1.5). The skin crease height is controlled by where the aponeurosis inserts and its depth is a feature of the levator function and state of the aponeurosis. If the aponeurosis stretches or disinserts the skin crease rises as in a ptosis caused by an aponeurotic weakness. If the skin crease is very shallow or virtually absent the levator function is likely to be very poor. If the patient is a young child with a significant ptosis a very shallow or absent skin crease increases the need for vigilance to avoid amblyopia.

The amount of eyelid which is visible when the person looks straight ahead in the primary position of gaze is called the upper lid show (Fig 1.6). It is controlled by the height and depth of the skin crease and the extent of the upper lid skin fold (Figs 1.5, 1.6). The skin fold consists of skin and preseptal orbicularis muscle with a possible protrusion of the preaponeurotic fat pad. With age there is a tendency for the skin crease to relax and become less deep, the brow becomes lower and together these contribute to an increased skin fold and decreased upper lid show. This can be improved with cosmetic surgery (Chapter 12) which aims to correct one or more of these factors i.e. (i) to raise the brow; (ii) reduce the skin, orbicularis muscle and possibly fat in the skin fold; and (iii) to reform the skin crease to hold the excess tissues away from the eyelid margin.

Skin fold

Brow level
Upper lid show

Lower lid skin crease

Figure 1.6

BROW LEVEL (Figs 1.1, 1.5, 1.6)

The brow is elevated by the frontalis muscle (Fig 1.1d) and depressed by the orbital orbicularis muscle (Fig 1.1c), corrugator (Fig 1.1q) and procerus muscle (Fig 1.1r). The brow level can be estimated by measuring the distance between the lid margin and the lowest brow hairs with the patient in the primary position of gaze (Fig 1.6). An estimate of the amount of skin in the upper lid can be obtained by making these same measurements with the patient looking down (Fig 1.5). The corrugator and procerus muscles are responsible for the glabella 'frown' lines – the creases which, as with any muscle, form at right angles to the line of action of the muscle. They can be very effectively reduced by injections of botulinum toxin. This will allow the frontalis muscle to act unopposed and lift the brow. This so-called chemical brow lift effect can be further enhanced if the orbital orbicularis muscle is injected with botulinum toxin just above and temporal to the lateral brow hairs.

LOWER LID RETRACTORS (Figs 1.7, 1.8)

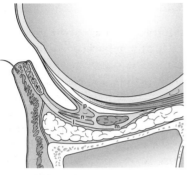

The lower lid retractors (Figs 1.3l, 1.7l) are responsible for the downward movement of the lower eyelid on downgaze. They consist of a sheet of fibrous tissue which extends from the sheath of the inferior rectus muscle, splits to enclose the inferior oblique muscle where it blends with the inferior suspensory (Lockwood's) ligament of the globe (Fig 1.7m), and runs forward to the lower border of the tarsal plate accompanied by some slips of smooth muscle – the inferior tarsal muscle (Fig 1.7n). This fibrous tissue sheet is analogous to the aponeurosis of the levator muscle, and the smooth muscle is analogous to the superior tarsal (Müller's) muscle (Fig 1.8). Laxity of these lower lid retractors contributes to entropion in the same way as an aponeurotic weakness of the upper lid causes ptosis.

Figure 1.7

SUSPENSORY LIGAMENT OF THE FORNIX
(Figs 1.4, 1.7)

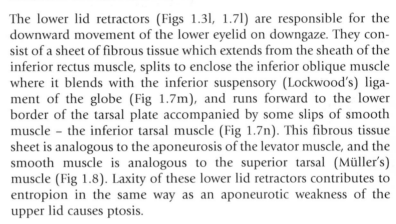

The fibrous tissue of the common sheath between the superior rectus and levator muscle continues forward as the superior suspensory ligament of the fornix (Fig 1.4o). If this is cut, e.g. during ptosis surgery, the conjunctiva can prolapse. The management is discussed in the section on complications of ptosis surgery.

In the lower lid the inferior suspensory ligament of the fornix is similarly part of the fibrous tissue of the lid retractors (Fig 1.7p). If these retractors are lax, e.g. involutional entropion, the lower fornix will tend to be shallow.

TARSAL PLATE

Figure 1.8

The tarsal plates consist of dense fibrous tissue. They form the skeleton of the lids, giving the lid margin stability. Provided that the tarsal plate is healthy, this stability can be maintained with only 4 mm of tarsus. The upper tarsal plate is usually 10–11 mm high and the rest of the upper tarsus can be used as a graft or tarsoconjunctival flap, as will be discussed under lid reconstruction. The lower tarsal plate should be used since it is only 3–4 mm high.

The tarsal plates contain the meibomian glands which open through the tarsal plate immediately posterior to the grey-line. This marks the separation between conjunctiva, which covers the tarsal plate, and squamous epithelium, which covers the orbicularis at the lid margin. An early sign of entropion is the anterior migration of the conjunctiva which occurs when the lid margin begins to invert and more of it comes into contact with the tear film (see severity of entropion, p 42).

MEDIAL CANTHAL TENDON

The medial canthal tendon is the tendon of insertion of the pretarsal and preseptal muscles. Like them, it has a superficial part which inserts onto the anterior lacrimal crest and a deep part which inserts onto the posterior lacrimal crest. The anterior limb can be divided without malposition of the medial canthus provided that the posterior limb remains intact. It is important to attempt to reform the posterior limb in any medial canthal reconstruction.

LATERAL CANTHAL TENDON

The lateral canthal tendon is the tendon of origin of the pretarsal muscles. It arises from a tubercle (Whitnall's) which lies 2 mm posterior to the lateral orbital rim. In any repair it is important to try and maintain one limb of the lateral canthal tendon to support and hold the reconstructed lid posteriorly against the globe. If both limbs are lost, the reconstructed lid or lids can be held posteriorly with sutures passed through a burr hole in the lateral orbital wall or with a periosteal flap reflected from the anterolateral orbital wall.

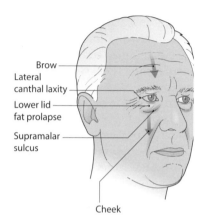

Brow
Lateral canthal laxity
Lower lid fat prolapse
Supramalar sulcus
Cheek

Figure 1.9

AGEING CHANGES IN THE FACE (Figs 1.9 and 1.10)

With ageing there is a generalised stretching and laxity of all the eyelid and facial connective tissues and muscles. The brows and cheek both become lower. This contributes to the appearance of excess tissue in the upper lids which is aggravated by laxity of the skin crease and stretching of the upper lid tissues themselves. In the lower lid when the cheek drops the nasojugal fold becomes more prominent and a relative hollow appears over the inferior orbital margin, the so-called supramalar sulcus or 'tear-trough' deformity. This is accentuated by any lower lid fat prolapse above the sulcus giving the appearance of 'dark circles' below the lower lids. The orbicularis muscle and medial and lateral canthal tendons stretch causing lower lid laxity, lid retraction and inferior scleral show. The increased laxity allows a greater movement of the eyelid tissues with an increase in the creases and wrinkles (rhytides) at right angles to the

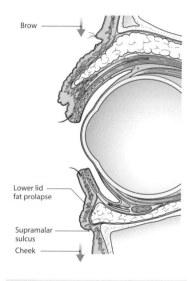

Brow
Lower lid fat prolapse
Supramalar sulcus
Cheek

Figure 1.10

orbicularis muscle action. The lower facial and neck tissues also drop aggravating the whole appearance of ageing.

Most of these changes can be improved with cosmetic surgery (Chapter 12) which aims primarily to reposition tissues and correct the effects of excess tissue laxity. This, however, will not correct the ageing changes in the skin itself which primarily affects the sub-epidermal tissues with collagen breakdown and elastosis aggravated by sun damage. Laser resurfacing, retinoic acid creams, etc. may be able to help reverse some of these skin changes but are beyond the scope of this book.

BLOOD SUPPLY

The lids are richly supplied by palpebral arteries formed by anastomoses between the internal and external carotid artery systems. This good blood supply is responsible for the rapid healing of eyelid wounds and the relative lack of infection. In the upper lid there are two main palpebral arcades, one on the tarsus and one lying over the lower part of the superior tarsal (Müller's) muscle. In the lower lid the palpebral artery lies on the tarsus usually 2–4 mm from the lid margin. It should not be cut by a horizontal lid transection provided that this is kept 4–5 mm below the lid margin.

ANAESTHESIA

The sensory supply of the eyelids is via the ophthalmic and maxillary divisions of the fifth nerve, the main supply being the supraorbital and infraorbital nerves. The supraorbital nerve can be blocked by feeling the supraorbital notch and passing a needle immediately below it, and through the orbital septum. Do not inject more than 1–2 ml of local anaesthetic or the levator muscle may be anaesthetised. The infraorbital nerve can be blocked by a local infiltration around the infraorbital foramen, which lies below the orbital rim approximately in line with the supraorbital notch. It is usually only necessary to use these nerve blocks to supplement local infiltration when deep surgery is undertaken. Local infiltration anaesthesia should be given immediately under the skin and conjunctiva to anaesthetise the nerve endings. The needle should preferably not enter the deeper tissues as this increases the risk of haemorrhage.

SUGGESTED FURTHER READING

1. Tyers AG, Collin JRO. A Colour Atlas of Ophthalmic Plastic Surgery. 2nd edn. Oxford: Butterworth Heinemann; 2001.
2. Chen, WP. Oculoplastic Surgery: The Essentials. New York: Thieme Medical Publishers; 2001.

3. Della Rocca RC, Bedrossian Jr EH, Arthurs BP. Ophthalmic Plastic Surgery: Decision Making and Techniques. New York: McGraw-Hill; 2002.
4. Leatherbarrow B. Oculoplastic Surgery. London: Martin Dunitz; 2002.
5. Levine MR. Manual of Oculoplastic Surgery. 3rd edn. Philadelphia: Butterworth-Heinemann; 2003.
6. Nerad JA. Oculoplastic Surgery: The Requisites in Ophthalmology. St. Louis: Mosby; 2001.
7. Olver J. Colour Atlas of Lacrimal Surgery. Philadelphia: Butterworth-Heinemann; 2004.
8. Katowitz JA. Paediatric Oculoplastic Surgery. New York: Springer-Verlag; 2002.
9. Chen WP, Khan JA, McCord CD. Colour Atlas of Cosmetic Oculofacial Surgery. Philadelphia: Butterworth-Heinemann; 2004.
10. Putterman AM. Cosmetic Oculoplastic Surgery: Eyelid, Forehead and Facial Techniques. 3rd edn. Philadelphia: Saunders; 1999.

Basic techniques

2

SUMMARY

This chapter summarises the basic techniques which are relevant to eyelid surgery including the principles of wound healing and suturing, technique of closing a full-thickness eyelid defect, how to take full-thickness or partial-thickness skin grafts for eyelid and socket reconstruction, what types of posterior lamella grafts are available and how to harvest them. What is meant by a middle lamella graft or implant and what tissues can be used to correct such defects. The principles of flaps and how they are used are discussed under lid reconstruction.

- Sutures and wound healing
- Closure of full thickness eyelid defects
- Anterior lamella grafts
- Posterior lamella grafts
- Middle lamella grafts

SUTURES AND WOUND HEALING
(Figs 2.1, 2.2, 2.3, 2.4, 2.5)

When tissues are injured with a surgical incision or as a result of other trauma the clotting mechanism and an inflammatory response is initiated. Fibrin is produced and the shape of the initial fibrin matrix influences how the wound eventually heals. This is why traction sutures are used in the first 24 hours to leave an eyelid over corrected after eyelid malposition surgery such as when lowering an upper lid (p 196) or raising a lower lid (p 200).

Wounds heal by either primary intention when the wound edges are apposed and the healing process occurs across the whole wound at the same time or by secondary intention when the wound is allowed to granulate and heal slowly from the base to the surface of the wound. The aim of most surgery is to create as fine a scar as possible. This is achieved by obliterating any dead space and by approximating the wound edge throughout the wound as accurately as possible using buried absorbable sutures to support the deep tissues and skin sutures to support the skin edges. Where the wound lies

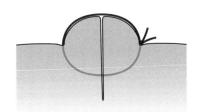

Figure 2.1

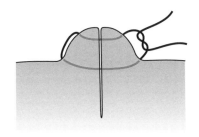

Figure 2.2

9

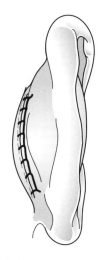

Figure 2.3

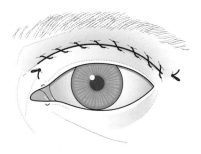

Figure 2.4

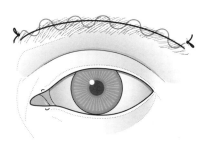

Figure 2.5

across the line of the underlying muscle or is under tension as in the repair of a pentagonal resection of full-thickness eyelid tissue, the skin edges need to be everted to compensate for the contraction of the wound tissues as they heal. This can be achieved by interrupted sutures (Fig 2.1) or double everting sutures (Fig 2.2). A locked running suture (Fig 2.3) is useful over a wider area such as closing a skin donor site after taking a graft from behind the ear (p 12). Wounds in the line of the underlying muscle such as in the skin crease are not under tension and only need to be gently approximated as with a running suture (Fig 2.4).

Fibroblasts very rapidly migrate into the wound and by 10 days the collagen that they form supports the wound and starts to contract. Most sutures can be removed at or by 10 days postoperatively although non-tension-bearing sutures such as a 'running suture' can be removed much earlier i.e. after about 5 days. The longer skin sutures are left the greater the risk of creating visible suture marks. This is usually only a significant risk when using interrupted sutures in forehead or thick eyelid skin where they should not be left for more than about 4 days. It is usually preferable to close forehead skin wounds with buried absorbable sutures and a continuous subcuticular suture (Fig 2.5) reinforced with steristrips if necessary. These must be placed across the line of the wound if they are going to support it effectively.

The phase of contraction in wound healing lasts about 12 weeks. During this period clinically there is some redness and thickening of the wound which is a normal physiological occurrence but needs to be explained to the patient especially in cosmetic cases such as following a blepharoplasty. Wound healing may be helped a little if vitamin E is applied to the wound postoperatively. If the wound becomes excessively red and thickened, local steroids either applied topically or in severe cases injected into the wound may help resolution as may pressure dressings, silicone dressings and massage etc. In situations where an excess cicatricial reaction can be anticipated, as with keloid scars, antimetabolites and other wound healing modulators can be tried.

Following surgery for the correction of eyelid malposition if, as the wound contracts, the ptosis or lid retraction starts to become a little over corrected, the wound can be stretched with eyelash traction and/or lid massage to counteract the wound contraction. This may be required for three minutes three times a day or as often as two minutes every two hours while the overcorrection persists. It may need to be continued for more than 12 weeks until the wound enters the phase of maturation and active contraction ceases. If the overcorrection persists after this, formal corrective surgery may be required as detailed in the chapters on ptosis surgery and thyroid lid retraction etc.

Although it is often desirable to reduce the active contraction phase of the wound healing it can be put to good use as when a wound is allowed to heal by planned secondary intention. This is called the laissez-faire technique which can be very useful for postir-radiation medial canthal defects (p 136) and for the exenterated socket (p 144). The open healing wound contracts, stretching the surrounding tissues and the surface of the wound epithelises.

CLOSURE OF FULL THICKNESS EYELID DEFECT (FIG 2.6)

Indications

A full thickness eyelid defect should be closed in two layers. If a full thickness eyelid resection is carried out it should be shaped as a pentagon so that when the tarsal plate is sutured together there is an even distribution of tension across the wound. If the resection was carried out as a wedge there would be maximum tension at the lid margin with the potential risk of causing a notch.

Method

1. Pass an absorbable suture on a half circle needle between the tarsal plate and orbicularis muscle and take a partial-thickness bit of tarsus about 1–2 mm from the cut edge and as near to the lid margin as possible. On the other side of the wound enter the tarsus near the conjunctival surface and bring the suture out between the tarsal plate and orbicularis muscle as on the first

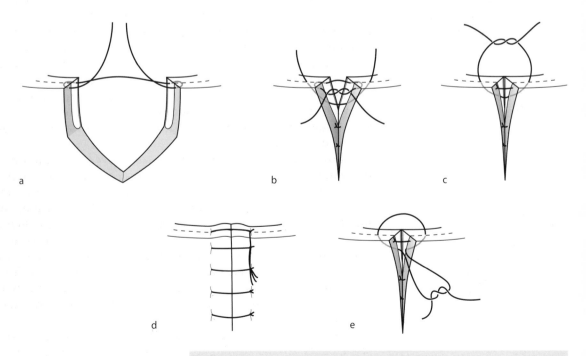

Figure 2.6

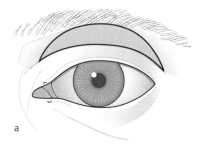

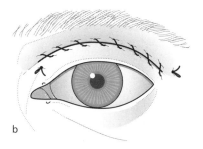

Figure 2.7

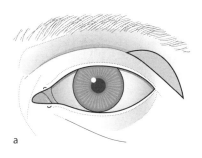

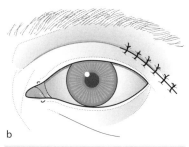

Figure 2.8

side (Fig 2.6a). Put a single throw in the suture and approximate the cut edges. Check the alignment of the lid margin and replace the suture if necessary.

Note: in the upper lid the suture must be buried in the tarsus to prevent a corneal abrasion, but it can be full-thickness through the tarsus in the lower lid.

2. Place two more absorbable sutures through the tarsal plate and tie them. Traction on the first suture will maintain the correct alignment and reduce haemorrhage.
3. Pass a 6 '0' silk suture through the grey-line and leave it loose (Fig 2.6b), then tie the uppermost absorbable suture (Fig 2.6c).
4. If the orbicularis muscle retracts beyond the wound edges, close it with an absorbable suture.
5. Tie the grey-line suture and leave the ends long.
6. Place a skin suture in the lash line, tie it, and leave the ends long.
7. Close the skin with interrupted sutures and catch the long ends of the previous two sutures in the uppermost knot. This prevents the suture ends from abrading the cornea (Fig 2.6d).
8. If there is an excessive amount of tension, place a 4 '0' nonabsorbable horizontal mattress suture across the wound and tie it over bolsters on either side of the suture line.
9. Remove the skin sutures at 5 days but leave the lid margin, lash line and uppermost skin suture for 10 days.

Note: 6 '0' long-acting absorbable sutures can be used instead of silk sutures and should be removed as described for silk sutures. If it is desirable to leave the sutures to absorb e.g. in a child, the lid margin sutures can be buried leaving only the segment of the suture at the grey-line exposed across the wound (Fig 2.6e).

ANTERIOR LAMELLA GRAFTS

A full thickness skin graft is preferable to a split thickness graft for closing anterior lamella defects of both lids unless not enough full thickness skin is available, e.g. in burns, or the graft bed is unfavourable, e.g. periosteum as when relining an exenterated socket.

SKIN GRAFTS

- Full thickness
- Split thickness

FULL THICKNESS SKIN GRAFT (Figs 2.7, 2.8, 2.9)

Indication

Skin replacement.

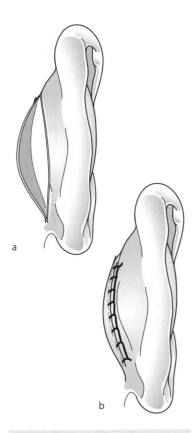

a

b

Figure 2.9

Donor sites

Upper lid skin above the skin crease (Fig 2.7), or laterally below eyebrow which is slightly thicker skin and less likely to limit eyelid closure (Fig 2.8), postauricular (Fig 2.9), supraclavicular fossa, inner arm, etc.

Method

1. Measure the defect.
2. Mark the donor site and check that it can be closed, e.g. if upper lid skin is to be taken hold the proposed donor skin in forceps and see that the lids can still close.
3. Excise the skin as thinly as possible. A subcutaneous injection of saline with or without epinephrine reduces the bleeding by tamponade and makes a graft easier to cut.
4. Close the donor site. A continuous pull-out or interrupted sutures can be used for the upper lid (Figs 2.7b, 2.8b) and removed at about 5 days. A 4 '0' nylon continuous locking suture can be used for the ear and should be left for 10 days (Fig 2.9b)
5. Excise the fat from the graft. There is no subcutaneous fat in upper lid skin, which improves its take as a graft.
6. Tailor the graft to fit the defect. Small perforations can be cut in a large graft to reduce the risk of a haematoma collecting under it. Suture the graft in place and hold it in contact with its bed. Interrupted 5 '0' black silk sutures can be used. If the ends are left long they can be tied over a bolster and the dressing left undisturbed for 5 days.

A better host/graft junction is usually achieved if a fine continuous suture is used to hold the graft accurately in place and a simple, slightly moist pressure dressing is applied for 48 hours without tie-over sutures. If there is any sign of a haematoma when the dressing is removed, it can be aspirated with a wide-bore needle and the dressing reapplied for a further 24 or 48 hours.

If early 'mobilisation' of the lids is essential the graft can be held against its bed by 'quilting', i.e. passing multiple interrupted sutures through the graft into the subgraft tissue (see Fig 3.14d, 'quilting' of the mucosal graft).

SPLIT THICKNESS SKIN GRAFTS

Indication

Skin replacement when not enough full thickness skin is available.

Donor sites

Inner arm or thigh.

Method

1. The graft can be taken with a split thickness skin knife or dermatome. If a split thickness skin knife is to be used preset the blade to cut the desired thickness of skin.
2. Lubricate the knife with KY Jelly.
3. Get the assistant to put the skin on tension.
4. Use a suitably shaped skin graft board to present the width of skin graft required.
5. Press the knife flat against the skin.
6. Cut the graft with a forward and backward motion of the blade advancing it until the desired length of graft has been obtained.
7. Cover the donor area with a sterile dressing. Leave it for 10 days and allow it to granulate.
8. Stretch the defect to a maximum with lid sutures to allow for subsequent shrinkage of the graft.
9. Suture the graft over the edge of the defect with interrupted sutures which are left long and used to tie over a pressure dressing.
10. Keep the lid on traction for 5 days, then remove the pressure dressing with all the sutures and trim off the excess skin.

POSTERIOR LAMELLA GRAFTS

I. Eyelid tissue
II. Mucosal lined tissue
a. oral
b. nasal
III. Nonmucosal lined tissue
a. autogenous
b. nonautogenous

I. EYELID TISSUE

It is always preferable to replace conjunctiva and tarsus with the same tissue if it is available i.e. 'replace like with like.'

a. Conjunctiva
b. Tarsus
c. Tarsomarginal graft

CONJUNCTIVA

Indication
Conjunctival deficit.

Donor site
Superior bulbar surface, inferonasal fornix.

Method

1. Inject local anaesthetic with epinephrine under the conjunctiva.
2. Cut around the proposed graft with a blade while the tissue is elevated with the local anaesthetic fluid.
3. Cut the subconjunctival tissue with spring scissors and slide the graft onto a spatula to keep it orientated correctly.
4. The superior bulbar surface can be allowed to granulate and heal by secondary intention. A 7 '0' absorbable suture can be used to close an inferonasal conjunctival defect.

TARSUS (Fig 2.10)

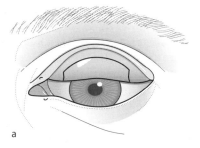

a

Indication

Tarsal deficit.

Donor site

Upper border of tarsus.

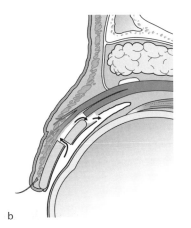

b

Figure 2.10

Method

1. Place a traction suture in the upper lid and evert it over a Desmarres' retractor.
2. Mark the desired graft size on the tarsus extending down from the attached upper border but leaving not less than 4 mm of intact tarsus to maintain the stability of the upper lid margin.
3. When satisfied with the extent of the graft and position of the donor site, make scratch incisions in the tarsus first and then cautiously deepen them to extend through the tarsus. If the lid is being forcibly everted the tarsal wound springs open when the tarsus is first cut through. The incision can then be completed with scissors along the scratch incisions.
4. If the tarsal graft is being used to reconstruct a lid margin leave a frill of conjunctiva attached to the tarsal graft.
5. Leave the donor site to granulate and heal by secondary intention. If the graft is small the donor eyelid level is not usually affected but if the graft is very extensive the lid level may rise unless the lid retractors are cautiously recessed via the posterior approach (p 196).

TARSOMARGINAL GRAFT (Fig 2.11)

Indications

Lid margin deficit.

Donor site

One or more of the three remaining uninvolved eyelids.

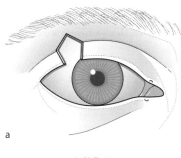

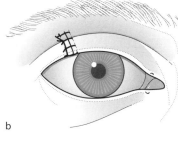

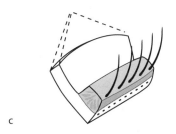

Figure 2.11

Method

1. Make a full thickness incision through the chosen donor eyelid starting at the junction of the lateral quarter with the medial three-quarters of the lid.
2. Extend the incision through the attached border of the tarsus.
3. Overlap the cut edges of the lid to assess how much lid can be removed and still allow the resulting defect to be closed directly. Excise up to this amount of full thickness eyelid (Fig 2.11a).
4. Close the donor site (p 11) (Fig 2.11b).
5. Excise the skin and orbicularis from the graft leaving about 3 mm of skin above the lashes (Fig 2.11c). This provides a tarsal graft with a stable eyelid margin. The eyelashes usually do not survive. More than one tarsomarginal graft can be joined together to reform the posterior lamella.

II. MUCOSAL LINED TISSUE

A full thickness oral mucous membrane graft is the simplest posterior lamella replacement graft to use if conjunctiva or tarsus is not available. A split thickness mucosal graft contracts more than a full thickness graft and is therefore less suitable for most eyelid and socket reconstruction. It should however be used on the globe where the graft is visible since a full thickness graft tends to look pink and bulky. Hard palate grafts are the stiffest oral mucosal grafts and contract the least. They are a little more difficult to harvest than other mucosal grafts but are useful when it is particularly desirable to avoid contracture e.g. raising the lower lid to correct thyroid lid retraction (p 200). Oral mucosa does not contain goblet cells and therefore does not supplement the tear film.

1. Oral
   a. Full thickness labial or buccal mucosa.
   b. Split thickness labial mucosa.
   c. Hard palate.
2. Nasal mucosa
   a. Turbinate
   b. Nasal septal cartilage and mucoperichondrium.

1. ORAL MUCOSAL GRAFTS

FULL THICKNESS ORAL MUCOSAL GRAFT

Indications

Posterior lamella or moist socket lining deficit.

Donor site

Lower or upper lip (labial), cheek (buccal).

Method

1. Measure the defect and cut an approximate template e.g. out of paper.
2. Place it on the chosen donor site. For the lip do not extend too close to the lip margin or gum. For the cheek adjust its position to avoid the opening of the parotid duct, usually opposite the second upper molar.
3. Make an incision peripheral to the template.
4. Inject saline under pressure to elevate the graft from the submucosal tissues and to reduce haemorrhage by tamponade. Weak epinephrine can be added to the saline but should not be necessary.
5. Excise the graft as thinly as possible using a blade and scissors.
6. Remove all the submucosal fat from the graft. This is easy if the graft is spread over the index finger, held by the thumb, and the fat excised with curved Westcott scissors.
7. The graft bed can be left to granulate or sutured with a few interrupted absorbable sutures if the defect is not too extensive.
8. Postoperatively cover the patient with systemic antibiotics. Mouth washes, fluids and a soft diet may be required initially, but the wound heals rapidly. It is rare to get any contracture but if necessary the cheek can be stretched by sucking marbles.

SPLIT THICKNESS MUCOUS MEMBRANE GRAFT

Indication

Conjunctival deficit especially on bulbar surface.

Donor site

Lip.

Method

1. Evert the lower lip and inject as much saline as possible under the mucosa to separate it from the submucosal tissues.
2. Use a mucotome, a small split-skin knife (e.g. Silver), or disposable dermatome, and excise approximately a 0.3 mm thickness of mucosa, taking care to avoid the vermilion border of the lip.
3. Leave the terminal part of the graft attached and remove the instrument. Slide a flat spatula under the graft and then cut off the terminal attachment. This ensures that you know which is the cut surface. If in doubt it is in theory possible to see which of the two surfaces stains with fluorescein, but this test is usually not very convincing.

4. Cauterise major bleeding points. Postoperatively the wound heals rapidly but cover the patient with systemic antibiotics and give mouth washes for the first few days.

Note: split thickness mucosa contracts but takes well on the lid margin. It produces the best cosmetic result when a visible conjunctival replacement graft is required on the globe.

HARD PALATE MUCOSAL GRAFT (Fig 2.12)

Indication

A stiff posterior lamella replacement.

Donor site

Hard palate.

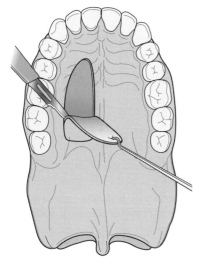

Figure 2.12

Method

1. Protect the teeth and hold the mouth wide open with a specially designed clamp, e.g. Dingman, or with dental or maxillofacial wedges or oral clamps.
2. Make a template of the defect and position this on the hard palate on one or other side of the midline raphe. Avoid the most anterior mucosa above the incisors and the mucosa over the roots of the molar teeth. Do not extend posteriorly onto the soft palate (Fig 2.12).
3. Incise around the edge of the template.
4. Inject local anaesthetic with epinephrine under the graft preferably using a dental syringe with a fine needle and a cartridge with 1 in 80 000 epinephrine.
5. Raise the corner of a posterior edge of the graft with a long handled toothed forceps and gently undermine the graft using a combination of a long handled blade alternating with a scleral pocket knife, angled keratome or beaver blade. Try to keep the resection as superficial as possible.
6. Remove any fat from the graft as with a full thickness mucous membrane graft.
7. Ensure haemostasis by cauterising the bed of the donor site.
8. Postoperatively cover the patient with systemic antibiotics. Mouth washes, fluids and a soft diet may be required initially. Postoperative pain can be a problem and may be relieved by sucking anaesthetic lozengers but these may also delay healing. A dental plate can be made to protect the site and allow healing to occur more quickly and comfortably. Postoperative haemorrhage is a risk. As a short-term measure the patient should be instructed to stick their thumb in their mouth over the donor site and apply pressure until it stops. Further cautery and systemic antibiotics may be required.

2. NASAL MUCOSAL GRAFTS

Grafts of nasal mucosa contain goblet cells which may contribute mucus to the tear film. This is maximised with turbinate mucosal grafts which can help to relieve discomfort in extreme dry eye situations. With nasal septal cartilage with its attached muco-perichondrium, the cartilage provides the skeleton for the lid replacing tarsus while the mucoperichondrium provides a mucosal lining which does not shrink. It can be wrapped around the skin of a reconstructed eyelid to form a stable eyelid margin.

NASAL TURBINATE MUCOSA (Fig 2.13)

Indication

Posterior lamella replacement requiring mucus producing goblet cells.

Donor site

Inferior turbinate.

Method

1. Decongest the nasal mucosa with a nasal pack containing a vaso-constrictor such as epinephrine.
2. Identify the inferior turbinate using a nasal speculum and a head light.

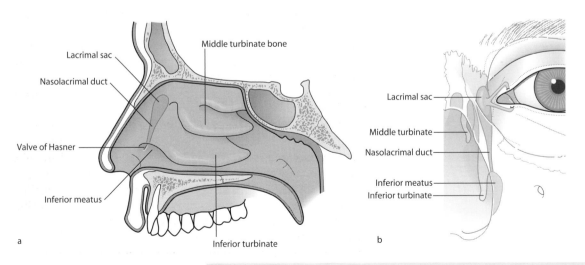

Figure 2.13

3. Slide a strong fine artery clamp around the base of the turbinate and firmly close the clamp.
4. Replace the clamp with scissors and excise the turbinate.
5. Spread out the turbinate mucosa on a moist gauze swab and remove the pieces of turbinate bone. The graft can then be sutured onto a suitable recipient site preferably hidden from view e.g. onto the bulbar surface above the superior limbus under the upper eyelid.
6. If there is bleeding, the nose can be packed for the first 24 hours. It is then treated with antibiotic and vasoconstrictor drops for about a month.

NASAL SEPTAL CARTILAGE AND MUCOPERICHONDRIUM (Fig 2.14)

Indication

A stiff posterior lamella replacement containing mucous producing goblet cells.

Donor site

The patient's nasal cartilage with the mucoperichondrium attached to one side. The other mucoperichondrium is left in situ.

Method

1. Reduce the vascularity of the septal mucosa preoperatively. In the anaesthetic room paint the nasal septum or pack the nose with a ribbon gauze soaked in a vasoconstrictor solution.
2. Use an operating headlight.
3. Give an extensive submucosal injection of a weak epinephrine solution on one side of the nose to help strip the mucosa from the cartilage.

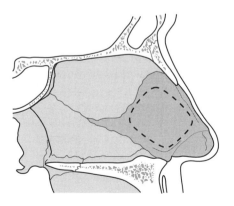
a
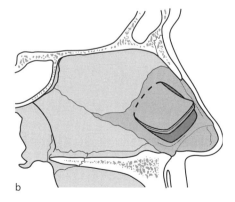
b

Figure 2.14

4. On the other side of the nose inject locally in the region of the planned incision only.

5. If adequate exposure cannot be obtained with a nasal speculum, cut around the alar base and lift the nostril.

6. Palpate the distal edge of the septum and incise through the mucosa proximal to and in line with it.

7. Clean the surface of the cartilage and partially cut through it with a blade, leaving a strut of septum to support the tip of the nose. Perforate the septal cartilage carefully with a blunter instrument such as a Rolletts rougine and push the mucoperichondrium away from the far side of the incision.

8. Complete the stripping of the mucoperichondrium with a periosteal elevator, e.g. a MacDonald.

9. Cut the cartilage and its attached mucosa with a specially designed 'swivel knife' if one is available. Alternatively, cut it from the roof and floor of the nose with scissors. Protect the stripped intact mucoperichondrium with a periosteal elevator.

10. If a swivel knife is not available, cut the proximal part of the septum and mucosa with an angled beaver blade, ground down keratome, scleral pocket knife or angled scissors.

11. Cut two fingers from a surgical rubber glove, pack them lightly with ribbon gauze, dip the fingers in glycerine and pack one finger on either side of the remaining mucoperichondrium. Remove the pack the following morning and treat the nose with antibiotic and vasoconstrictor drops four times a day for about a month.

    Note: The septal cartilage usually requires thinning before it is used.

III. NONMUCOSAL LINED GRAFTS AND IMPLANTS

Various tissues which do not have a mucosal lining can be used as posterior lamella grafts. They depend on conjunctivalisation i.e. conjunctiva growing over the surface of the graft. These may be autogenous grafts, e.g. cartilage, or nonautogenous, e.g. sclera, or a scleral substitute, e.g. Alloderm. Since these grafts do not have a mucosal lining they can also be buried within the tissues to act as a spacer to hold the lid retractors recessed, as in treatment of lid retraction (p 196). They can also be buried within the tissues to stiffen the lid, e.g. auricular cartilage as an upper lid sandwich graft (p 49). Sclera was used extensively for such purposes as there was a plentiful supply from corneal graft banks and it avoided the need to harvest an autogenous graft. However, it is now much less popular because of the potential risk of transmitted disease such as HIV and Creutzfeldt-Jacob.

a. Autogenous:
   – ear cartilage.

b. Nonautogenous:
   – sclera
   – sclera-like substitutes e.g. Alloderm

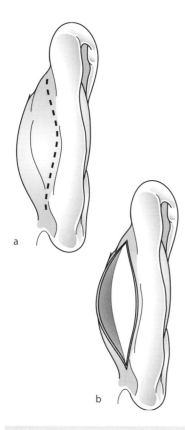

Figure 2.15

EAR CARTILAGE GRAFT (Fig 2.15)

Indication

A stiff posterior lamella which can conjunctivalise; a middle lamella spacer or stiffener of a reconstructed eyelid.

Donor site

The flattest part of the helix.

Method

1. Mark the main concavity of the helix on the posterior surface of the ear (Fig 2.15a).
2. Inject local anaesthetic and epinephrine solution subcutaneously under the mark. This is difficult because the tissues are tightly adherent to the cartilage. A dental syringe with a fine needle may be helpful.
3. Cut through the skin mark to the cartilage on the posterior surface of the ear.
4. Separate the subcutaneous tissues from the cartilage either centrally towards the skull (Fig 2.15b) or towards the edge of the ear. Cartilage can be taken from either or both sides of the main curve in the cartilage but this should be left intact to maintain the shape of the ear.
5. Cut partially through the cartilage with a knife and complete the incision with a blunter instrument like a Rolletts rougine. This reduces the risk of perforating the whole ear. Free the cartilage from the anterior layer of perichondrium and excise it.
6. Obtain haemostasis and suture the skin with a continuous locking 4 '0' nylon suture. A fine rubber drain can be sutured into the wound if it is difficult to control the bleeding. Alternatively pressure can be applied by suturing a pressure dressing to itself on each side of the ear across the donor site using 4 '0' nylon or similar sutures.
7. The ear should be carefully padded with wool. Postoperative swelling is marked. If a drain is used it should be removed at 24–48 hours and the nylon suture at 10 days.

SCLERA

Indication

As a posterior lamella graft which will conjunctivalise with time; a middle lamella graft or spacer to lengthen or recess the lid retractors; as a cover for a buried orbital implant.

Origin

Donor eye.

Method

1. Take a donor eye which has been harvested and probably used for corneal grafting.
2. Excise the remnants of Tenon's capsule, the extraocular muscles and the optic nerve.
3. Evaginate the scleral shell over a finger and remove all the intraocular contents and uvea.
4. Clean the uveal surface with a dry swab.
5. Store the scleral shell in 70% alcohol in the refrigerator.
6. Wash it thoroughly in saline with several changes of solution over the 24 hours prior to use.
7. Soak it in an antibiotic solution 2 hours prior to use.
8. Rinse it in saline and cut it to the required shape.

ALLODERM

Indication

Posterior lamella graft which will conjunctivalise; middle lamella graft.

Origin

Human dermis in which the proteins have been denatured and the tissue freeze dried and sterilised.

Method

Open the packet and follow the instructions which include hydrating the Alloderm and removing the tape prior to use.

It is wise to use a marker pen to mark the side from which the tape has been removed so that the Alloderm is correctly orientated when sutured into position.

MIDDLE LAMELLA GRAFTS AND IMPLANTS

The middle lamella is a useful concept when considering eyelid reconstruction. It can be thought of as everything between the anterior lamella of skin and the posterior lamella of conjunctiva and tarsus. Middle lamella grafts may be required if there is no shortage of skin or conjunctiva but the lid is retracted e.g. thyroid lid retraction when the lid retractors may need to be lengthened with a 'spacer' such as sclera, ear cartilage or Medpor. Alternatively a lid may be retracted with scar tissue after trauma when a dermis fat graft may be required. Other examples include an upper lid ptosis or lax lower lid which may need to be raised or supported with a sling of fascia or other material. A reconstructed lid margin may be unstable if there is no middle lamella and an ear cartilage graft can be used to stiffen it as a sandwich between the anterior and posterior lamella. Some of these grafts can also be used as posterior lamella grafts and allowed to conjunctivalise as described above. Manufactured implants such as mersilene mesh, Gortex, Medpor or hydroxyapatite can be used to supplement the 'middle lamella' but must be well buried within the tissues.

I. Autogenous
  a. Fascia lata
  b. Dermis fat
  c. Ear cartilage
II. Nonautogenous
  a. Homologous:
    – Sclera
    – Alloderm
  b. Manufactured:
    – Mersilene mesh
    – Gortex
    – Medpor
    – hydroxyapatite

AUTOGENOUS MIDDLE LAMELLA GRAFTS

FASCIA LATA (Fig 2.16)

Indications

Frontalis sling/brow suspension ptosis surgery; lower lid fascial sling; autogenous wrapping material for implants; middle lamella spacer.

Donor site

Outer side of leg.

Method

1. Make a 3–4 cm vertical skin incision above the knee joint in a line between the head of the fibula and the anterior iliac crest (Fig 2.16a).
2. Separate the subcutaneous fat with large blunt-ended scissors until the deep fascia is exposed.
   Note: the required fascia is a glistening sheet of white vertically running collagen fibres. If this is not seen it is likely that the fascia has been exposed too anteriorly where it is thinner and more irregular in direction.
3. Clean the fascia and make two vertical incisions through the fascia about 1 cm apart.
4. Separate the fascial strip from its deep attachments to the underlying muscle with a pair of curved artery forceps (Fig 2.16b).

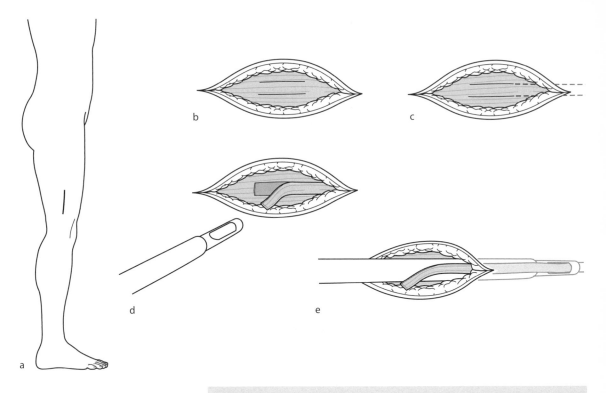

Figure 2.16

5. Extend the two vertical splits in the fascia subcutaneously up the thigh by splitting along the line of the collagen fibres with long-handled scissors held partially open (Fig 2.16c).
6. Cut the lower end of the fascial strip and introduce it into a fascial stripper (e.g. Crawford, Masson, Mustardé) (Fig 2.16d).
7. Cut the upper end of the fascia with the fascial stripper which is passed up the thigh around the strip of fascia (Fig 2.16e).
8. Close the subcutaneous fat with interrupted 3 '0' long-acting absorbable sutures and the skin with a subcuticular 4 '0' nylon suture which is left for 10 days. Do not close the fascia directly as this can lead to postoperative discomfort. Apply a firm dressing around the thigh for 48 hours.
9. Clean the strip of fascia and split it into appropriately sized strips e.g. approximately 3 mm wide for frontalis sling/brow suspension ptosis surgery and a little wider for a lower lid fascial sling (p 108 and 219). Keep them moist.

Complications

Muscle hernia. This is relatively rarely a significant problem but if a repair is required the hernia can be reinforced with materials such as Mersilene mesh.

DERMIS FAT GRAFT (Fig 2.17)

Indications

Primary or secondary autogenous orbital implant, especially after trauma; replacement of extruding implant; orbital volume replacement when lining is also required as in a volume-deficient contracted socket; deep upper lid sulcus correction despite orbital floor implant and orbital implant if appropriate; middle lamella graft to correct scarring or volume deficit.

Donor site

Buttock, lower abdomen.

Method

1. (a) Mark a banana-shaped ellipse on the buttock skin in the area covered by the underpants and not immediately over the ischial tuberosity. The centre of the ellipse should allow a 25 mm disc of dermofat to be removed and the ends should be curved to follow the flexion of the buttock (Fig 2.17b).

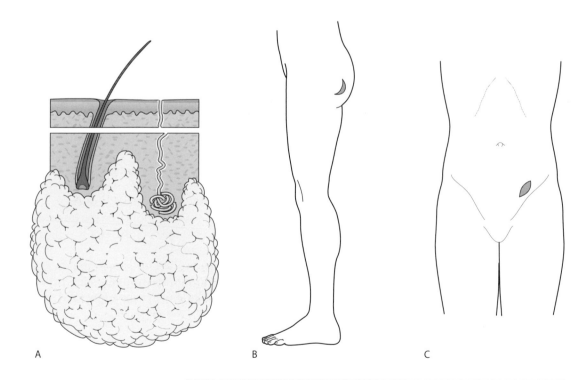

A   B   C

Figure 2.17

(b) The abdomen provides a good alternative donor site although less fat may be available if the patient is thin. Mark an elipse on the left lower abdomen. Avoid the right side as the scar might be confused with an appendicectomy scar. (Fig 2.17c)

2. Make a fine scratch incision through epidermis only.
3. Inject saline under pressure with a 10 ml syringe and a fine-bore needle into the epidermis to create a 'peau d'orange' appearance.
4. Shave the epidermis with a sharp scalpel blade (no. 10 or 15). Fat globules will be exposed if the cut is too deep and epidermis will be left behind if it is too shallow.
5. Cut through the dermis into the fat to a depth of about 25 mm, but stop if the deep fascia over the buttock muscles is encountered before this.
6. Remove the graft and suture the deep fat and dermis in layers using a 4 '0' long-acting absorbable suture with a large needle.
7. Close the skin with 4 '0' nylon sutures.
8. Support the wound with Elastoplast or similar tape for 4–5 days.
9. Remove the sutures after 10 days.
10. After taking a dermis fat graft from the buttock encourage showers for the next 3–4 weeks rather than sitting in a hot bath to reduce the risk of wound dehiscence.

Complications

Unsightly scar; wound dehiscence. If this occurs a useful technique is to soak a swab in Chlorhexidine and Cetrimide solution. Apply the swab to the open wound for 5 to 10 minutes once or twice a day. Cover the wound with a light, dry gauze dressing and allow it to granulate and heal by secondary intention which may take several weeks.

MANUFACTURED MIDDLE LAMELLA IMPLANTS

MERSILINE MESH, GORTEX, MEDPOR, HYDROXYAPATITE

Indications

Middle lamella implants which become vascularised and integrated to various degrees within the tissues can be used to raise the upper lid in ptosis surgery or support a lower lid (Mersilene mesh, Gortex); push up a lower lid (Medpor) or correct a volume deficit etc.

Origin

Manufactured.

Complications

Any manufactured material which becomes integrated and vascularised can cause granulomas if the tissue becomes exposed. It may then need to be removed. Autogenous materials are therefore usually preferable but do need to be harvested.

Entropion and trichiasis

3

ENTROPION

In entropion the eyelid margin turns inward against the eye. The anterior lamella of the eyelid consists of skin and orbicularis muscle and the posterior lamella of tarsus, conjunctiva and the lid retractors. For an entropion or ectropion to occur there must be a relative dissociation of the lamellae.

CLASSIFICATION

Congenital
– Epiblepharon
– Entropion
Acquired
– Involutional
– Cicatricial

CONGENITAL EPIBLEPHARON/ENTROPION

AETIOLOGY

At birth the anterior and posterior lid lamellae are often not clearly adherent i.e. they are relatively dissociated. The orbicularis muscle is well developed and there is a tendency for a fold of skin and orbicularis in the medial part of the eyelid to push the eyelashes toward the eye causing an epiblepharon. This is common in Asian races. It often cures itself as the child gets older and the lamellae become more adherent to each other. If the changes are more severe the whole eyelid margin inverts, causing an entropion.

SYSTEM FOR EPIBLEPHARON/ CONGENITAL ENTROPION

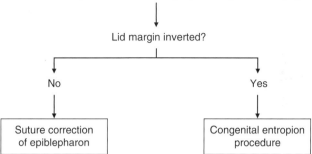

Lashes abrading cornea and causing significant persistent symptoms

Lid margin inverted?

No → Suture correction of epiblepharon

Yes → Congenital entropion procedure

SUTURE CORRECTION OF EPIBLEPHARON
(Fig 3.1a,b)

Principle

Sutures are passed from below the tarsal plate and tied on the apex of the epiblepharon fold of skin to hold the two lamellae together.

Indications

Epiblepharon which does not resolve in the first two years of life and causes eyelashes to abrade the cornea producing recurrent attacks of conjunctivitis.

Method

1. Pass about three double-armed 4 '0' long-acting absorbable sutures from below the lower border of the tarsal plate and tie them on the skin over the apex of the epiblepharon fold (Fig 3.2a,b).
2. Remove these sutures after about three weeks or leave them to absorb of their own accord.

Complications

If the sutures are left to fall out of their own accord they may bury themselves under the skin and set up an abscess as they absorb. If the sutures start to bury themselves or become infected try to remove them and give systemic antibiotics.

CONGENITAL ENTROPION PROCEDURE (Fig 3.2)

Principle

An ellipse of skin and orbicularis muscle is excised from below the inferior punctum. The skin edges are sutured to the lower lid retractors and lower border of tarsus (Hotz-type operation).

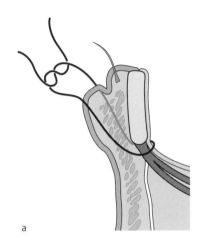

a

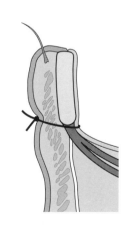

b

Figure 3.1

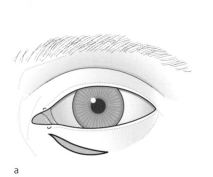
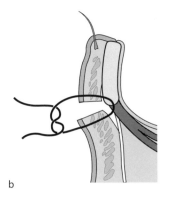
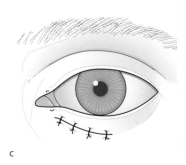

a   b   c

Figure 3.2

Indications

Frank lower lid entropion with inversion of the lid margin in a child who is persistently photophobic and gets recurrent attacks of conjunctivitis which do not resolve in the first two years of life.

Method

1. Use forceps to pick up the minimum excess skin and orbicularis muscle which just corrects the entropion. Mark this as an ellipse in the medial part of the eyelid.
2. Excise the ellipse of skin and orbicularis muscle (Fig 3.2a).
3. Suture the lower lid skin edges to the retractors and lower border of the tarsal plate with interrupted long-acting 6 '0' absorbable sutures (Fig 3.2b).
4. Do the procedure bilaterally to create a symmetrical scar (Fig 3.2c).
5. Leave the sutures to fall out spontaneously.

Complications

It is very easy to excise too much tissue and create an ectropion in later life.

ACQUIRED LOWER LID ENTROPION

This is either involutional and due to ageing changes or cicatricial and due to any condition that causes conjunctival scarring e.g. trauma, chemical burns, trachoma, infection (especially chronic staphylococcal blepharoconjunctivitis), pemphigoid, Stevens-Johnson syndrome etc.

SYSTEM FOR ACQUIRED LOWER LID ENTROPION

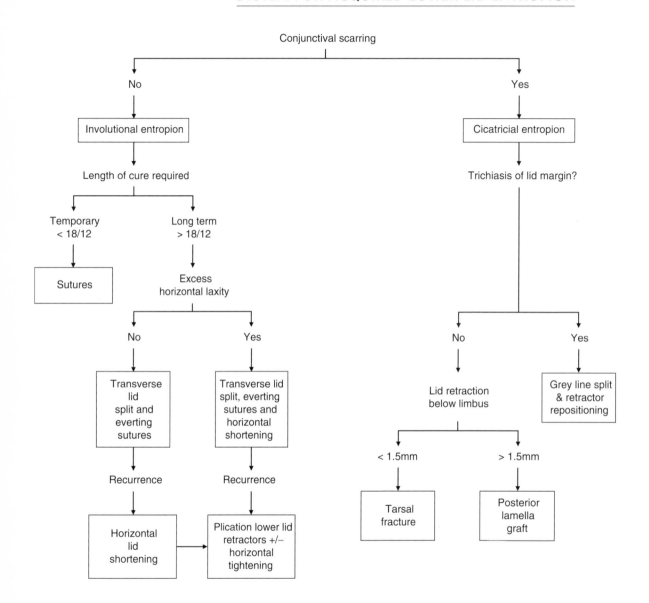

INVOLUTIONAL ENTROPION

PATHOPHYSIOLOGY OF EYELID AGEING CHANGES

Ageing changes in the eyelid are similar whether they cause entropion or ectropion. Laxity of tissues causes lamella dissociation or slippage of the anterior lamella over the posterior lamella. In entropion the anterior lamella and preseptal orbicularis muscle moves upwards. This is a fundamental cause of involutional entropion. In ectropion there is a relative upward movement of the posterior lamella. In both entropion and ectropion the lower lid retractors become lax and no longer control the inferior border of the tarsal plate. In ectropion they may become frankly disinserted, causing the lid to evert as a shelf and allowing the conjunctiva to become oedematous. In entropion and ectropion the orbicularis muscle with its medial and lateral canthal tendons becomes relaxed and the tarsus itself may stretch, causing increased horizontal lid laxity. This may be aggravated by some enophthalmos of the globe. Secondary changes occur in the tarsus which in entropion becomes thin and buckled.

The main ageing changes which require correction in both involutional entropion and ectropion can be summarised as follows:

- Lamella dissociation
- Lower lid retractor weakness
- Horizontal lid laxity.

AETIOLOGY AND MANAGEMENT OF INVOLUTIONAL ENTROPION (Fig 3.3)

1. **Lamella dissociation** (upward movement of preseptal muscle)
   Treatment: Create a scar tissue barrier between the preseptal and pretarsal muscles with transverse sutures or transverse lid split etc.
2. **Lower lid retractor weakness**
   Treatment: Tighten retractors with everting sutures, plication or shortening of lower lid retractors.
3. **Horizontal lid laxity**
   Treatment: Shorten the lid and/or canthal tendons.
4. **Buckling of tarsal plate**
   Treatment: Everting sutures to transfer pull of lower lid retractors to evert the lid margin.

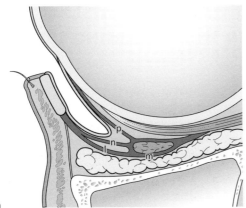
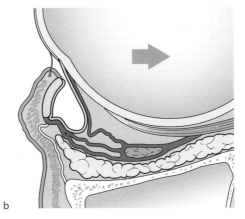

Figure 3.3

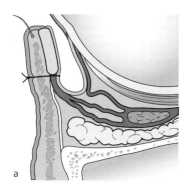

a

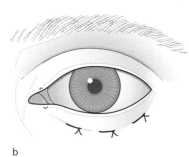

b

Figure 3.4

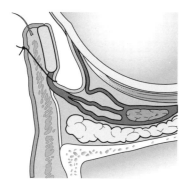

Figure 3.5

SUTURES (Figs 3.4, 3.5)

Principle

Sutures can be used to correct the lamella dissociation either as (1) transverse sutures to prevent the upward movement of a preseptal muscle (Fig 3.4) or as (2) everting sutures to tighten the lower lid retractors and evert the lid margin (Fig 3.5).

Indications

Temporary cure (up to 18 months or longer) with a quick, easy, repeatable procedure which can be performed at the bedside, e.g. geriatric patient, following ocular surgery, waiting for definitive entropion correction etc. Use transverse sutures if the entropion mainly occurs when the patient forcibly closes the lid and there is an element of spasm. Everting sutures are often used as part of other entropion procedures.

Method

Pass three double-armed 4 '0' long-acting absorbable sutures through the lid from the conjunctiva to the skin in the lateral two-thirds of the lid. With transverse sutures start just below the tarsus, pull the preseptal skin downwards and make each needle emerge through the skin about 2 mm apart and just above the level at which they entered the conjunctiva (Fig 3.4). Everting sutures are similar but start lower in the fornix and emerge nearer to the lashes (Fig 3.5). Tie the sutures tightly and remove them after 2–3 weeks.

Complications

Recurrences will occur but sutures can be a useful temporary procedure. A more permanent operation aims to correct more of the aetiological factors.

TRANSVERSE LID SPLIT + EVERTING SUTURES (WIES-TYPE PROCEDURE) (Fig 3.6)

Principle

The lid is split transversely to create a fibrous tissue scar barrier which prevents the upward movement of the preseptal muscle. This is combined with everting sutures which shorten the lower lid retractors and transfer their pull to the upper border of the tarsus.

Indications

'Long-term' cure (more than 18 months) of an entropion with little horizontal lid laxity.

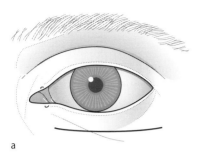

a

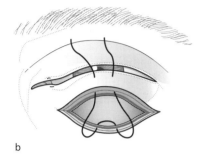

b

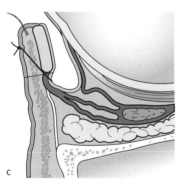

c

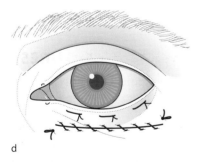

d

Figure 3.6

Method

1. Make a horizontal skin incision 4 mm below the lash line and a little lower laterally (Fig 3.6a).
2. Protect the globe with a lid guard.
3. Perforate the lid with sharp pointed scissors at the medial and lateral ends of the skin incision.
4. Cut horizontally through the whole lid along the line of the skin incision. Take care to keep the scissors horizontal so that the conjunctiva and skin are cut at the same level. The incision is made 4 mm below the lash margin to avoid cutting the tarsal plate.
5. Identify the lower lid retractors, which are visible as a layer of white fibrous tissue lying just anterior to the conjunctiva. They should be seen and felt to move downwards when the patient looks down. If necessary, the inferior fat pad can be exposed with blunt dissection behind the preseptal orbicularis muscle. The lower lid retractors lie between the fat pad and the conjunctiva.
6. Pass three double-armed 4 '0' long-acting absorbable sutures from the conjunctiva below the lid transection to the skin above it. Each needle should enter the conjunctiva about 2 mm apart and 2 mm below its cut edge, pass through the lower lid retractors, cross the lid transection, pass between the tarsal plate and the pretarsal muscle, and emerge through the skin 1–2 mm below the lash line (Fig 3.6b).
7. Close the skin with a continuous or interrupted sutures.
8. Tie the double-armed sutures under enough tension just to evert the lid margin. Start with the lateral suture and avoid a punctal ectropion when the medial suture is tied (Fig 3.6c,d).
9. Remove the skin sutures at 5 days. The everting sutures should be removed at 10–14 days or earlier if there is a marked overcorrection.

Complications

Recurrence is usually due to the existence or more lid laxity than was appreciated preoperatively. It can be corrected by horizontally tightening the lid.

Overcorrections can be caused by tightening the everting sutures too much. This can be corrected by early suture removal. If the overcorrection persists the lid must be reoperated and the lamellae dissociated before the lid is reconstituted with less aggressive everting sutures.

TRANSVERSE LID SPLIT, EVERTING SUTURES + HORIZONTAL LID SHORTENING (QUICKERT PROCEDURE) (Fig 3.7)

Principle

The transverse lid split prevents the upward movement of the preseptal orbicularis, the everting sutures shorten the lower lid retractors and transfer their pull to the upper border of the tarsus, and the

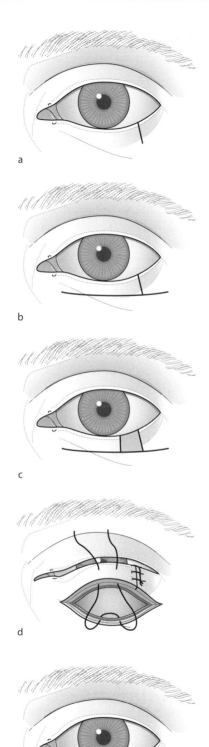

horizontal lid shortening corrects the excess lid laxity and prevents the lid turning in or out.

Indications

'Long-term' cure (more than 18 months) of an entropion with excess horizontal lid laxity assessed by pulling the lid away from the globe.

Method

1. Make a 'vertical' incision through the lid from the lid margin to the lower border of the tarsal plate, starting 5 mm from the lateral canthus (Fig 3.7a).
2. Make a horizontal full-thickness lid incision just below the tarsal plate to the inferior punctum medially. Keep the scissors horizontal to cut the skin and conjunctiva at the same level.
3. Make a similar incision laterally which keeps horizontal and does not follow the contour of the lid margin (Fig 3.7b).
4. Identify the lower lid retractors and place three double-armed 4 '0' long-acting absorbable sutures through them and the conjunctiva, starting about 2 mm below the transection.
5. Overlap the two flaps of eyelid to assess the extent of the lid resection necessary to compensate for the excess horizontal laxity. Resect this amount from the medial flap (Fig 3.7c).
   Note: if the excision of this amount of tissue would displace the lower punctum excessively, the medial canthal tendon should be plicated first to stabilise it (see p 63). The excess horizontal laxity should then be reassessed and the lid resected as before.
6. Suture the two flaps of eyelid as in a normal lid repair (see p 11).
7. Pass the double-armed 4 '0' long-acting absorbable sutures in front of the tarsal plate, and behind the pretarsal muscle, and emerge through the skin 1–2 mm below the lash line (Fig 3.7d). Then continue as from stage 6 of the transverse lid split and everting sutures procedure (Fig 3.7e).
8. If there is excess skin and muscle below the horizontal lid transection the skin can be undermined, pulled laterally as for a blepharoplasty, and the excess skin excised as a base-up lateral triangle (see Fig 12.7).
9. Remove the skin sutures at 5 days but leave the lid margin and everting sutures for 10 days.

Complications

Recurrence is usually due to failure to shorten the lower lid retractors adequately and can be corrected with a lower lid retractor plication type of procedure.

Overcorrection is caused and treated in a similar way to that described for a 'transverse lid split and everting sutures'.

Figure 3.7

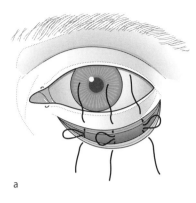

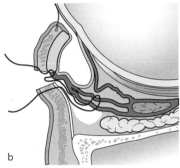

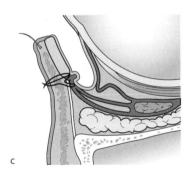

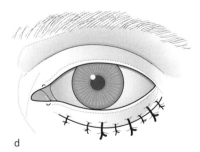

Figure 3.8

PLICATION OF LOWER LID RETRACTORS (JONES TYPE PROCEDURE) (Fig 3.8)

Principle

The lower lid retractors are exposed via a skin approach, shortened, and the sutures used to create a barrier to the upward movement of the preseptal muscle.

Indications

As a primary entropion procedure coupled with horizontal lid tightening if indicated or for recurrent entropion, e.g. after transverse lid split, everting sutures and lid shortening. Such a recurrence is likely to be due to a lower lid retractor weakness since everting sutures will not adequately tighten the retractors if they are excessively lax or disinserted.

Method

1. Make a horizontal skin incision at the lower border of the tarsal plate.
2. Separate the pretarsal and preseptal muscles to expose the inferior edge of the tarsal plate.
3. Dissect deep to the preseptal muscle and divide the inferior orbital septum. The orbital fat lies anterior to the lower lid retractors.
4. Retract the orbital fat and confirm that the lower lid retractors move up and down with movements of the globe.
5. Pass a 4 '0' long-acting absorbable suture through the lower skin edge in the centre of the lid, through the lower lid retractors about 8 mm below the tarsus, through the lower border of the tarsal plate, and out through the upper skin edge (Fig 3.8a,b).
6. Tighten this suture and tie it with a slip knot.
7. Observe the effect. The lid margin should be in a normal position and should move normally on up and down gaze. If there is an undercorrection replace the suture taking a lower, proximal bite of the retractors, and if there is an overcorrection replace it taking a higher bite nearer the tarsus.
8. When the correction is satisfactory, undo the knot and place 2–4 more similar sutures, 1–2 medial and 1–2 lateral to this central suture (Fig 3.8c).
   Note: a. The sutures can be left with a slip knot which can be loosened or tightened and tied 4–24 hours after surgery if required. These adjustable sutures are particularly helpful with recurrent entropions if it is difficult to set the lid confidently at the time of surgery.
   b. Excess skin and orbicularis muscle can be excised from the lower edge of the skin incision if required.
9. If the lid is lax tighten it.

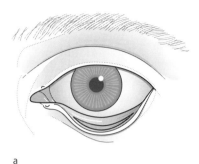

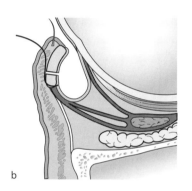

a

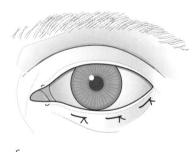

b

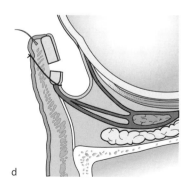

c

d

Figure 3.9

10. The skin closure is reinforced with interrupted 6 '0' sutures preferably identified by a different colour. These are placed between the retractor plicating sutures (Fig 3.10d). This allows the plicating sutures to be removed early if they are causing over-correction.
11. Skin sutures can be removed at 7 days and the plicating sutures at 14 days

Complications

Overcorrection. Loosen or remove plicating sutures.
Undercorrection. Tighten sutures if they are adjustable or redo operation.
Recurrence. Assess the likely causes and re operate aiming to correct them.

LOWER LID CICATRICIAL ENTROPION

TARSAL FRACTURE (Fig 3.9)

Principle

The tarsus is fractured horizontally and hinged into eversion with everting sutures.

Indications

Mild cicatricial entropion in which the cicatrisation has not caused the lid margin to be retracted by more than about 1.5 mm below the limbus.

Method

1. Make a horizontal incision through the whole width of the tarsal plate just below its centre (Fig 3.9a).
2. Expose the deep surface of the pretarsal muscle but do not carry the incision through the skin and orbicularis as there would be a risk of inducing necrosis of the lid margin with such a high incision.
3. Free the anterior tarsal surface from the pretarsal muscle and continue this lamella dissociation to free the lower lid retractors and orbital septum from the preseptal muscle so that the lid margin can evert.
4. Pass three double-armed 4 '0' long-acting sutures just below the lower fragment of the tarsal plate and out through the skin immediately below the lash line (Fig 3.9b).
5. Tie these everting sutures tightly deliberately to overcorrect the entropion. Allow the tarsal fracture and 'hinge' to granulate (Fig 3.9c,d).
6. Remove the sutures at 2–3 weeks. As the scar contracts, the lid margin will be pulled back against the globe.

Complications

Insufficient eversion of the lid margin. A more effective but more complex way of everting the lid margin is with a grey-line split and lower lid retractor repositioning procedure, but this may increase lid retraction.

Recurrence of the entropion with lid retraction requires a posterior lamella graft.

POSTERIOR LAMELLA GRAFT (Fig 3.10)

Principle

The tarsoconjunctiva is lengthened with a graft inserted near the lid margin to allow eversion.

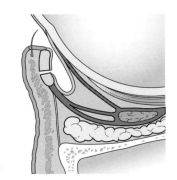

a

Indications

Severe cicatricial entropion; entropion with lid retraction of more than about 1.5 mm below the limbus; recurrence of entropion after tarsal fracture procedure.

Method

1. Pass 2 × 4 '0' nonabsorbable traction sutures through the grey-line to evert the lid.
2. With traction on these sutures, evert the lid over a Desmarres' retractor and make a transverse incision through the tarsal plate (Fig 3.10a).
3. Free the inferior edge of the tarsal plate, the orbital septum and lower lid retractors from the orbicularis muscle and allow the posterior lamella to retract.
4. Free the anterior surface of the upper fragment of tarsus to allow it to evert completing the lamella dissociation. N.B. This often results in cutting the traction suture which will then need to be replaced.
5. Take a full thickness posterior lamella graft of e.g. buccal or hard palate mucosa, tarsal plate, ear cartilage or Alloderm etc. and suture it between the cut edges of the tarsal plate. A continuous 6 '0' absorbable suture or 5 '0' nylon pull out suture can be used.
6. Hold the lid margin everted and the graft against its bed with two or three 4 '0' long-acting absorbable sutures passed through the graft and tied on the skin just below the lashes (Fig 3.10b)
7. Remove these sutures at 5–10 days.

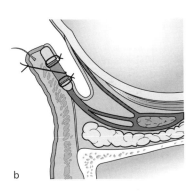

b

Figure 3.10

Complications

Overcorrection and eversion of the lid margin is often due to the lid being too lax. This may require to be corrected with a horizontal tightening procedure.

Undercorrection is usually due to an inadequate posterior lamella graft. A further graft is usually required.

GREY-LINE SPLIT AND RETRACTOR REPOSITIONING (Fig 3.11)

Principle

The lid margin is split at the grey-line. The lower lid retractors are attached to the anterior lamella just below the lashes to forcibly evert the split lid margin.

Indications

A moderately severe cicatricial entropion with trichiasis but without significant lid retraction, especially where it is undesirable to make an incision in the tarsus or conjunctiva such as in ocular cicatricial pemphigoid.

Method

1. Evert and stabilise the lower lid with a finger.
2. Identify the meibomian gland orifices. Make an incision immediately in front of them and behind any area of trichiasis or aberrant eyelashes.
   Note: the lower lid is thin and it is difficult to achieve this cut without damaging the roots of the lashes.
3. Deepen the grey-line split incision to a depth of 2–3 mm.
4. Make an incision through the skin and orbicularis muscle 3–4 mm below the lid margin. Open the orbital septum and expose the lower lid retractors.
5. Free the lower border and anterior surface of the tarsus from the pretarsal orbicularis muscle.
6. Pass a 5 '0' double-armed long-acting absorbable suture into the lower lid retractors and bring each arm out in front of the tarsus and through the pretarsal orbicularis muscle just below the lash line (Fig 3.13a). Tie the two arms of the suture together with a bow knot. The grey-line split should open. If the sutures cause lid retraction they should be repositioned taking a bite of the lower lid retractors nearer to the lower border of the tarsus. If the grey-line split is not adequately everted clean the anterior surface of the tarsus more effectively and bring the sutures out closer to the lash line and/or take a lower bit of the lower lid retractors.
7. When the lid margin is adequately everted and the grey-line split opened widely without causing significant lid retraction, place another 2–3 sutures (Fig 3.11b).
8. Close the skin with a continuous 6 '0' nylon suture or interrupted sutures (Fig 3.11c). Apply an antibiotic ointment to the grey-line split about four times daily and allow it to granulate. Remove the sutures after about 2 weeks.

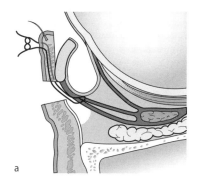

a

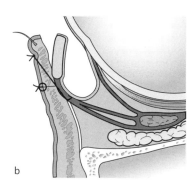

b

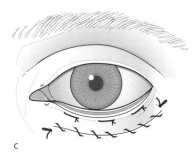

c

Figure 3.11

Complications

Lid retraction caused by placing the sutures too low in the retractors. They need to be removed and replaced.

Granuloma formation of the split everted lid margin. This usually recovers spontaneously.

Recurrence which may require a posterior lamella graft and/or more immunosuppression if appropriate e.g. if there is an exacerbation in ocular cicatricial pemphigoid.

UPPER LID ENTROPION

SYSTEM FOR UPPERLID ENTROPION

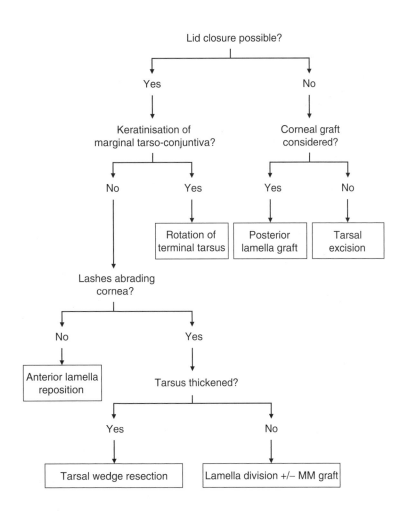

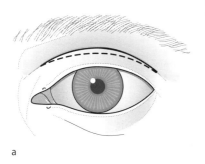

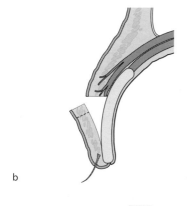

a

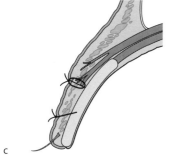

b

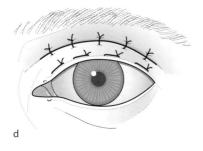

c

d

Figure 3.12

AETIOLOGY AND MANAGEMENT

Any cause of conjunctival scarring can lead to an upper lid entropion. The cicatrising process has various effects which influence the choice of operation:

- Severity of the entropion
- Thickness of the tarsal plate
- Keratinisation of the tarsal conjunctiva
- Lid retraction.

1. Severity of the entropion

If the cicatrisation is mild, lashes may not frankly abrade the cornea, but the early changes of entropion can be detected by the apparent posterior migration of the meibomian gland orifices and conjunctivalisation of the lid margin.

Treatment: Mild entropion: anterior lamella reposition.

2. Thickness of the tarsal plate

Cicatrising conditions like trachoma cause a thickened tarsal plate, while in other conditions, e.g. Stevens-Johnson syndrome, the tarsal plate may be thin. If the tarsal plate is thick it can be everted by cutting a wedge out of it, but this is impossible if the tarsal plate is thin.

Treatment:

Thick tarsal plate: tarsal wedge resection.

Thin tarsal plate: lamella division ± mucous membrane graft.

3. Keratinisation of the marginal tarsoconjunctiva

The cicatrising process may lead to metaplastic changes such as keratinisation and aberrant fine hair formation. If this occurs on the posterior surface of the tarsus near the lid margin, this area must be everted away from the cornea.

Treatment: Rotation of terminal tarsus.

4. Lid retraction

Any cicatrisation which causes an upper lid entropion shortens the posterior lid lamella. If this is mild it can be corrected by freeing the conjunctiva from Müller's muscle and any subconjunctival scar tissue, and advancing the posterior lamella of tarsoconjunctiva. This should be part of any upper lid entropion operation. If the lid retraction is so severe that the eyelids do not meet on forced lid closure, the posterior lamella must be lengthened with a graft and the lid margin everted, or the scarred tarsus must be excised and the conjunctiva and lid retractors recessed.

Treatment:

Mild retraction: advance tarsoconjunctiva and free Müller's muscle.

Severe retraction: posterior lamella graft or tarsal excision.

ANTERIOR LAMELLA REPOSITION (Fig 3.12)

Principle

The anterior lamella of skin and muscle is undermined, repositioned and sutured to the tarsus at a higher level. It is also sutured to the aponeurosis with the skin closure sutures. This increases the eversion and reforms the skin crease.

Indications

Mild upper lid entropion.

Method

1. Make an incision in the skin crease (Fig 3.12a).
2. Free the anterior tarsal surface until the lash roots are just visible (Fig 3.12b).
3. Pass a 6 '0' long-acting absorbable suture through the skin just above the lashes, into the tarsal plate at a higher level, and out through the skin again about 2 mm from and at the same level as it entered the skin.
   Note: a. The height of the tarsal fixation controls the lash eversion.
   b. If an adequate eversion of the lashes cannot be achieved by repositioning the tarsal fixation, the eversion can be increased by splitting the lid margin just anterior to the orifices of the meibomian glands to a depth of 1–2 mm (see Fig 3.13a). This split is allowed to granulate.
4. Excise the small excess of skin and muscle which is created by the repositioning.
5. Close the skin with interrupted 6 '0' absorbable sutures which pick up the aponeurosis (Fig 3.12c,d).
6. Remove the long-acting absorbable sutures after 6 weeks if they have not fallen out on their own. If they get infected they should be removed earlier.

Complications

Localised suture abscess. Treatment: remove offending suture.

TARSAL WEDGE RESECTION (Fig 3.13)

Principle

An anterior lamella reposition and lid margin split is combined with the excision of a wedge of tarsal plate.

Indications

Marked upper lid entropion with a thickened tarsus, no keratinisation of the marginal tarsoconjunctiva, and with the eyelids able to meet on forced lid closure.

Method

1. Evert the lid and make an incision 1–2 mm deep in the lid margin just anterior to the orifices of the meibomian glands (Fig 3.13a).
2. Make an incision in the skin crease (Fig 3.13b), and undermine the anterior tarsal surface until the lash roots are almost visible.

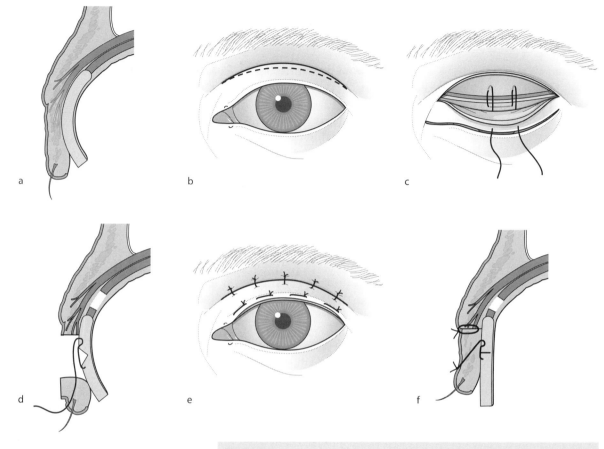

Figure 3.13

It is preferable to leave a bridge of tissue between the lid margin split and the exposure of the anterior tarsal surface.

3. With a blade, cut a wedge out of the anterior tarsal surface along the line of maximum tarsal thickening.

4. Dissect fibrous tissue and Müller's muscle off the upper border of the tarsal plate and conjunctiva sufficiently to advance the posterior lamella and compensate for the degree of lid retraction.

5. Close the tarsal wedge and evert the lashes with about four double-armed 6 '0' long-acting absorbable sutures. Pass a needle horizontally into the tarsal plate below the wedge and above the lash roots. Take each arm of the suture and with the needle pick up the tarsus above the wedge. Then pass each needle through the skin just above the lashes about 2 mm apart. Tie the sutures tightly. This closes the tarsal wedge, everts the lashes and opens the split in the lid margin (Fig 3.13c,d).

6. The rest of the procedure is the same as that for an anterior lamella reposition, stages 4–6 (Fig 3.13e,f).

Complications

Excessive eversion of the lid margin. Treatment: Early removal of sutures.

LAMELLA DIVISION ± MUCOUS MEMBRANE GRAFT (Fig 3.14)

Principle

The lid is split completely into an anterior lamella of skin and orbicularis and a posterior lamella of tarsus and conjunctiva. The posterior lamella is advanced and held in position with sutures passed through the lid. The raw anterior tarsal surface can be allowed to granulate but heals quicker if covered with a mucous membrane graft.

Indications

Marked upper lid entropion with a thin tarsus (Fig 3.14a), no keratinisation of the marginal tarsoconjunctiva, and with the eyelids able to meet on forced lid closure.

Method

1. Split the lid margin just anterior to the orifices of the meibomian glands and extend the split upwards to divide the lid into an anterior and posterior lamella.
2. Free the whole anterior surface of the tarsal plate and as much of the conjunctiva into the fornix as is necessary to advance the posterior lamella to compensate for any lid retraction (Fig 3.14b).
3. Pass three double-armed 4 '0' long-acting absorbable sutures from the upper fornix, through the conjunctiva, and out through the skin in the position of the prospective skin crease. Tie them. They should hold the posterior lamella advanced below the anterior lamella by about 4 mm.

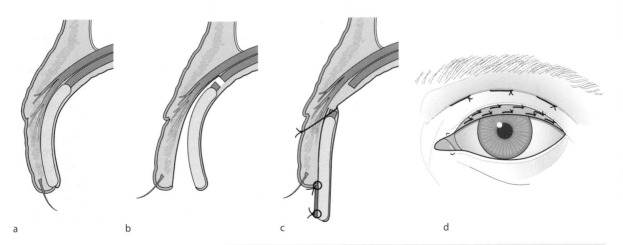

a   b   c   d

Figure 3.14

4. Suture the recessed edge of the anterior lamella directly to the advanced tarsus and evert the lashes. Leave the 4 mm of exposed raw surface to granulate, or suture a split-thickness (or thin full-thickness) mucous membrane graft to the raw anterior surface of the tarsus and to the free edge of the anterior lamella with multiple interrupted 6 '0' absorbable sutures (Fig 3.14c,d).
5. The 4 '0' long-acting absorbable sutures can be removed at 10 days.

Complications

If the recessed edge of the anterior lamella is not sutured to the tarsus, the resulting cleft may epithelialise. Treatment: Excision of epithelium and resuture.

ROTATION OF TERMINAL TARSUS (TRABUT TYPE PROCEDURE) (Fig 3.15)

Principle

The tarsus is cut and the lower portion rotated through 180°. The posterior lamella is advanced to make a new lid margin.

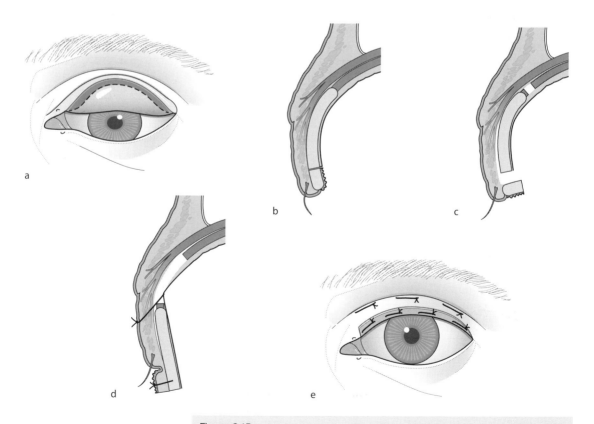

a

b

c

d

e

Figure 3.15

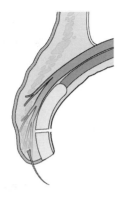

a

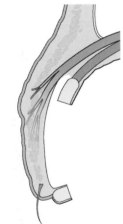

b

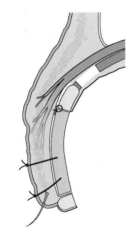

c

Figure 3.16

Indications

Upper lid entropion with metaplastic changes such as keratinisation and aberrant hair growth involving the lower posterior tarsal surface which is in contact with the cornea.

Method

1. Evert the lid and make an incision through the tarsus above the marginal strip of metaplastic change, i.e. normally 2–3 mm from the posterior lid margin (Fig 3.15a,b). The lid can be everted over a lid guard with skin hooks but it is easier to hold it with a Crookshank clamp or one of its modifications (e.g. Barrie Jones).
2. Free the anterior surface of the tarsal plate and the conjunctiva up to the fornix to allow the posterior lamella of the lid to advance freely.
3. Undermine the anterior surface of the lower distal tarsal fragment. Make a horizontal relieving incision through the lid margin at the lateral canthus and make a similar vertical incision immediately lateral to the upper punctum. Continue the undermining until the lower fragment of tarsus everts freely through 180° (Fig 3.15c).
4. Pass three double-armed 4 '0' long-acting absorbable sutures through the lid from the conjunctival surface of the upper fornix to the prospective skin crease. They should hold the posterior lamella advanced, and the anterior lamella with the attached distal fragment of tarsus recessed, so that the initial incision through the tarsus becomes the new lid margin.
5. Suture the everted fragment of tarsus to the anterior tarsal surface with interrupted 6 '0' long-acting absorbable sutures (Fig 3.15d,e).
6. The 4 '0' long-acting absorbable sutures can be removed at 10 days. The 6 '0' long-acting absorbable sutures are managed as in stage 6 of an anterior lamella reposition procedure.

Complications

Thickened lid margin. Treatment: This usually resolves after several weeks.

Loss of normal lashes. This is a significant risk but is usually acceptable if ocular discomfort has been significantly improved. It must be discussed with the patient preoperatively.

POSTERIOR LAMELLA GRAFT (Fig 3.16)

Principle

The tarsus is divided, the terminal fragment everted and a graft sutured between the everted terminal tarsal fragment and the recessed conjunctiva and lid retractors.

Indications

Entropion associated with severe upper lid retraction such that the lid margins will not meet on forced lid closure. A posterior lamella graft is essential if a corneal graft is considered in these circumstances.

Method

1. Make a horizontal incision in whatever remains of the tarsal plate (Fig 3.16a).
2. Free and evert the terminal tarsal fragment (Fig 3.16b).
3. Free the upper border of the tarsus and conjunctiva and recess the lid retractors to overcorrect the defective lid closure.
4. Suture a graft of preferably nasal septal cartilage with its attached mucoperichondrium or hard palate mucosa into the defect between the upper tarsal fragment and the everted lower fragment. Use buried 6 '0' long-acting absorbable sutures to suture it to the upper fragment. Suture it to the orbicularis muscle and lid margin with similar sutures tied on the skin (Fig 3.16c) or use 5 '0' long-acting absorbable sutures which can be tied over bolsters if preferred.

    Note: The graft should be stiff and mucosal lined. Contralateral tarsus is ideal but is seldom available. Ear cartilage is stiff but not mucosal lined. It can cause corneal problems. A mucous membrane graft can be used and the lid 'stiffened' later with a sandwich graft of ear cartilage (see p 49).

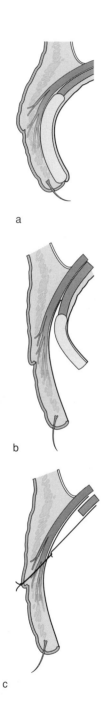

a

b

c

Figure 3.17

Complications

Corneal abrasions from the surgery, rough surface of nonmucosal lined grafts or keratinisation of the graft. Treatment: Protective contact lenses may be required.

TARSAL EXCISION (Fig 3.17)

Principle

The tarsus is excised and the conjunctiva and lid retractors are recessed and held with sutures passed through the lid. The raw posterior lid surface rapidly becomes conjunctivalised. If the tarsal remnant is excised the underlying fibrous tissue may cause less entropion. The improved comfort may be acceptable if no corneal graft is planned.

Indications

Entropion associated with severe lid retraction and a small scarred tarsus which cannot be everted (Fig 3.17a).

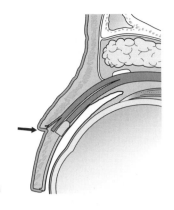

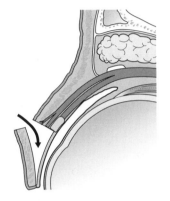

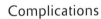

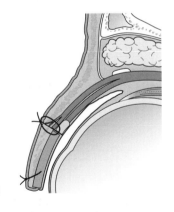

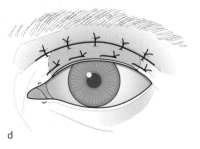

a

b

c

d

Figure 3.18

Method

1. Split the lid into an anterior and a posterior lamella (Fig 3.17b).
2. Free the conjunctiva and lid retractors extensively into the upper fornix.
3. Excise the tarsal remnant.
4. Pass three double-armed 4 '0' long-acting absorbable sutures through the lid to hold the conjunctiva and lid retractors recessed as far as possible (Fig 3.17c). These sutures can be left to absorb on their own or removed after 10 days.

Complications

Unstable lid margin and recurrence of entropion. Treatment: Formal lid margin and posterior lamella reconstruction.

AURICULAR CARTILAGE AS UPPER LID SANDWICH GRAFT (Fig 3.18)

Principle

Auricular cartilage is placed superficial to conjunctiva or tissue used to reconstruct the posterior lamella of the lid and deep to orbicularis muscle or skin as a 'sandwich graft' to stiffen the lid. If the graft is placed close to the reconstructed eyelid margin a stable eyelid margin can be achieved.

Indications

Unstable eyelid margin in reconstructed upper lid e.g. after Cutler-Beard lower lid bridge flap (p 130).

Method

1. Make an appropriate skin crease incision (Fig 3.18a).
2. Cut through the deep tissue to expose the posterior lamella (Fig 3.18b).
3. Dissect the posterior lamella as far as the reconstructed upper lid margin.
4. Take an auricular cartilage graft (p 22), clean off all the perichondrium and cut it to the desired size, e.g. to simulate an upper tarsus. If necessary make smaller partial thickness incisions in the tarsus to correct any aberrant curvature and get it to lie as required.
5. Place the prepared auricular cartilage graft over the cleaned posterior lamella, under the skin and orbicularis and as close to the lid margin as possible. Hold it in this position and evert the anterior lamella with 6 '0' long-acting absorbable sutures. Pass these through the skin just above the reconstructed lid margin, into the auricular cartilage at a higher level and out

through the skin again as anterior lamella repositioning sutures.

6. Reform the skin crease with 6 '0' long-acting absorbable sutures (Fig 3.18c,d).

7. As with any anterior lamella repositioning procedure, remove the long-acting absorbable sutures after 4 weeks if they have not fallen out before on their own. If they get infected they should be removed earlier.

Complications

Cartilage grafts can develop localised overgrowth of cartilage if the perichondrium has not been completely removed. Treatment. Reopen the wound and shave down the excess tissue.

SUMMARY OF SURGERY FOR UPPER LID ENTROPION

MILD

Anterior lamella reposition.

MODERATE/SEVERE

Thick tarsus: tarsal wedge resection.
Thin tarsus: lamella division ± mucous membrane graft.
Keratinisation of tarsoconjunctiva: rotation of terminal tarsus.
Lid retraction:
    moderate – posterior lamella advancement.
    severe – posterior lamella graft or tarsal excision.
Unstable reconstructed lid margin: auricular cartilage as sandwich graft.

TRICHIASIS

DEFINITIONS

- Aberrant lashes: normal position, abnormal direction.
- Distichiasis: second row of lashes from meibomian gland orifices.
- Metaplastic lashes: abnormal position.

MANAGEMENT OF ABERRANT AND MALPOSITIONED LASHES

Electrolysis, cryotherapy or surgical excision, or incision combined with electrolysis, cautery or cryotherapy are standard methods of treating trichiasis. Hair follicles can be destroyed in many other ways such as laser and radiotherapy and by various ingenious operations not covered in this book. Any entropion or other eyelid margin mal-position must be corrected with appropriate surgery, e.g. entropion or ectropion repair. The choice of procedure for trichiasis depends on the number and position of the lashes. A localised notch at the eyelid margin with trichiasis remains best treated with a simple full thickness lid resection but it is wise to subject any resected specimen to histology as such a notch may harbour unsuspected malignancy e.g. a basal cell carcinoma.

- Single (few) lashes – electrolysis
- Localised area of trichiasis
  - Confined to anterior lamella: anterior lamella excision
  - Full thickness notch: full thickness resection
- Many lashes – cryotherapy

ELECTROLYSIS

Principle

Passage of needle electrode down hair follicle to hair bulb which is destroyed by electric current.

Indications

Single or few malpositioned eyelashes.

Method

Give local anaesthesia and insert the chosen electrolysis needle down the hair follicle. Take care to be as accurate as possible and follow the manufacturer's instructions for the individual instrument chosen.

Complications

With any electrolysis there is approximately a 50% recurrence rate as it is extremely difficult to ensure that the needle does accurately reach and destroy only the hair bulb. If it goes through the hair follicle wall the electrolysis will not kill the hair bulb and will cause scarring which may distort adjacent hair follicles causing other eye-lashes to become malpositioned. Various modifications of instruments have been introduced to limit this complication such as insulation of the electrolysis needle leaving only the tip exposed, spring-loaded needles which in theory will pass down the hair follicle etc.

ANTERIOR LAMELLA EXCISION (Fig 3.19)

Principle

The lid is split at the grey-line. A small portion of the anterior lamella with all the lash roots is excised. The bare anterior surface of the tarsus

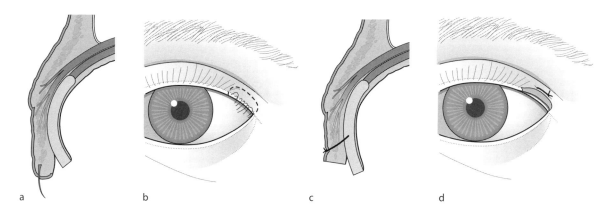

a   b   c   d

Figure 3.19

is cauterised to stop bleeding and destroy any eyelash roots which may have been left behind.

Indications

Aberrant eyelashes confined to a localised portion of the anterior lamella, e.g. lateral part of an eyelid.

Method

1. Give local anaesthesia or general anaesthesia if necessary e.g. children.
2. Split the grey-line behind the area of trichiasis to a depth of about 3 mm i.e. above the anticipated length of the hair bulb (Fig 3.19a).
3. Excise the area of the anterior lamella and cauterise the anterior tarsal surface (Fig 3.19b).
4. Place an anterior lamella repositioning or everting suture through the skin into the tarsus at a higher level and out through the skin just above the cut lower edge of the anterior lamella. This will partially evert the new lid margin and help to prevent a localised area of entropion or skin/globe contact when the raw anterior tarsal surface granulates and epithelialises (Fig 3.19c,d).

Complications

Ocular irritation from skin/globe contact and partial entropion in the treated area.

Treatment. Correct any true entropion. Excise skin in the area that has granulated and hold the cut edge of the anterior lamella more effectively recessed with a better placed anterior lamella repositioning suture.

CRYOTHERAPY

Principle

Lash follicles are more sensitive to the destructive effects of freezing than epithelial cells and connective tissue. The cryodestructive effect is enhanced by the rapidity of the freeze, the duration of the thaw, the number of freeze–thaw cycles, and various other factors. The object is to reduce the temperature at the follicles to about −20°C as quickly as possible, to allow the tissue to thaw as slowly as possible, and to repeat the freeze–thaw cycle. This can be achieved with various specially designed probes or with liquid nitrogen spray. The ordinary cryoprobe, such as is used in cataract or retinal surgery, is not capable of routinely achieving a low enough temperature. The appearance of the tissues when frozen is no guide to the actual temperature at the lash follicles and it is essential to monitor the temperature with a thermocouple. If a large series of patients has been monitored using the same technique and equipment, it is reasonable to use the average time taken in the series to achieve −20°C at the lash follicles and to dispense with the thermocouple.

Indications

Trichiasis or malpositioned eyelashes of any kind, e.g. aberrant lashes, distichiasis or metaplastic lashes when the eyelid margin is in the correct position and it has been agreed that destruction of all eyelashes both normal and abnormal is acceptable.

Method

1. Instill local anaesthetic drops into the conjunctival sac and infiltrate the lid with local anaesthetic preferably containing epinephrine.
2. Insert the thermocouple needle in the region of the lash follicles, deep to the orbicularis muscle and superficial to the tarsal plate.
3. Protect the globe with a non-metal lid guard if required (a plastic coffee spoon is effective). The surrounding tissues can be protected with tape if liquid nitrogen spray is used.
4. Freeze the lid from the skin surface with liquid nitrogen, or from either surface with a probe, to a monitored temperature of −20°C. Allow the tissues to thaw spontaneously to a positive temperature. Repeat the cycle.
5. Use an antibiotic ointment locally for 5–7 days. Postoperative swelling and even blistering of the skin can be quite marked but this is not uncomfortable after the first few hours as local nerve conduction is inhibited by the freezing.

Complications

Destruction of normal lashes. Various techniques have been described for trying to limit the extent of the ice ball so that it does not destroy the normal lashes but none of them are guaranteed and unless the patient is prepared to lose their normal lashes as well as the abnormal ones they should not undergo cryotherapy.

Depigmentation. This will occur because pigment cells are more sensitive to cold than lash follicles. It limits the use of cryotherapy in dark skinned patients although various techniques for limiting depigmentation have been described as discussed above. Re pigmentation may occur with time but cannot be guaranteed.

Thinning of eyelid. Cryotherapy does lead to thinning of eyelid tissues and may cause an unstable lid margin, particularly if the cryotherapy is repeated.

MANAGEMENT OF DISTICHIASIS

- Single/few lashes. Lash root exposure and direct destruction
- Many
  - Upper lid. Lamella division and cryotherapy to posterior lamella.
  - Lower lid. Cryotherapy.

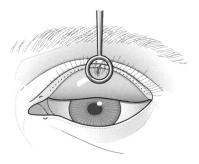

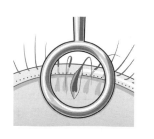

Figure 3.20

LASH ROOT EXPOSURE AND DIRECT DESTRUCTION (Fig 3.20)

Principle

The lash root or hair bulb can be exposed anywhere in the eyelid by making a small vertical cut through the eyelid tissues along the line of the hair follicle. Bleeding can be controlled with a meibomian clamp. The lid can be split at the grey-line to facilitate access to anteriorly placed abnormal eyelashes. The technique is particularly useful for distichiasis lashes which can be approached posteriorly through the everted tarsal surface. The hair bulb is destroyed by direct electrolysis or cautery. If the incision is partial thickness vertical and linear there is very little scarring and little risk of inducing an entropion or trichiasis from damage to adjacent lash roots.

Indications

Single or few distichiasis lashes. (It can be used for other aberrant lashes as indicated under 'principle'.)

Method

1. Evert the eyelid.
2. Place a meibomian clamp centred over the aberrant eyelash.
3. Make a partial thickness incision through the posterior lid margin to expose the aberrant eyelash.
4. Extend the cut to follow the shaft of the eyelash to its root i.e. the hair bulb. This is preferably carried out under the microscope (Fig 3.20).

5. Electrolyse or cauterise the lash root under direct vision. The vertical lid split will heal spontaneously.

Complications

The procedure is time-consuming if more than one or a few eyelashes need to be treated. Tarsal scarring, recurrence and entropion can occur if the hair follicle is not accurately exposed and destroyed.

LAMELLA DIVISION AND CRYOTHERAPY TO POSTERIOR LAMELLA (Fig 3.21)

Principle

The lid is split into an anterior and posterior lamella, keeping as close as possible to the tarsal plate to preserve the normal lashes. The posterior lamella is frozen to destroy the abnormal lashes. It is then advanced and the lid reconstituted, leaving the raw anterior surface of the tarsal plate to granulate.

Indications

Extensive distichiasis of upper eyelid.

Method

1. Follow stages 1 and 2 of the lamella division ± mucous membrane graft upper lid entropion procedure (see p. 45).
2. Freeze the terminal tarsus to −20°C with a double freeze–thaw cycle, monitoring the temperature with a thermocouple on the conjunctival surface of the tarsus (Fig 3.21b).
3. Pass through-the-lid sutures as in stage 3 of lamella division ± mucous membrane graft procedure.
4. Suture the anterior lamella to the tarsus with interrupted 6 '0' absorbable sutures, leaving approximately the lower 4 mm of the raw tarsal plate exposed and advanced (Fig 3.21c).

   Note: a. No mucous membrane graft is sutured to the anterior tarsus since it has been frozen.

   b. This procedure can be used equally well in dark-skinned people since the anterior lamella is not frozen so there should be no skin depigmentation.

   c. A similar procedure can be used in the lower lid in dark-skinned people. Depigmentation is prevented but the normal lashes are usually lost since it is very difficult to split the lower lid and preserve them.

Complications

Upper lid entropion. It is essential to advance the posterior lamella adequately to prevent contraction of the granulating tarsal plate leading to an upper lid entropion. If the patient does develop an

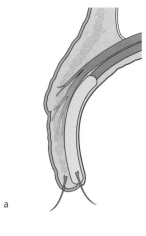

a

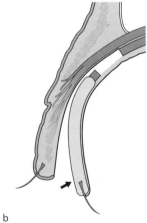

b

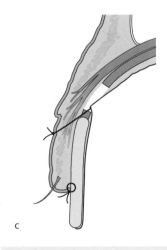

c

Figure 3.21

entropion it can be managed as any other upper lid entropion usually with a grey-line split and anterior lamella repositioning procedure.

Loss of normal eyelashes. The patient must be warned that however carefully the lid margin is split some or all of the normal lashes may be lost.

METAPLASTIC LASHES

Lid margin position normal: cryotherapy (for single or few lashes, electrolysis or lash root exposure and direct destruction of hair bulb can be tried).

Lid margin position abnormal: entropion procedure, usually rotation of terminal tarsus ± cryotherapy etc.

Ectropion

4

Ectropion is a condition in which the eyelid margin everts away from the globe.

CLASSIFICATION

- Congenital
- Acquired
  - involutional
  - mechanical
  - cicatricial
  - paralytic

CONGENITAL

- acute eversion
- congenital ectropion

ACUTE EVERSION

AETIOLOGY

In neonates the eyelid lamellae are not very tightly adherent. Orbicularis spasm can induce slippage or lamella dissociation leading to an acute eversion of the lid. This particularly occurs in premature infants.

TREATMENT

1. Manual repositioning and inversion of the lid plus antibiotic ointment.
2. If conjunctival oedema makes it difficult to keep the lid in the normal position with manual repositioning use inverting sutures (Fig 4.1a,b; see p 72).
3. Full thickness horizontal lid shortening and inverting sutures may very rarely be required.

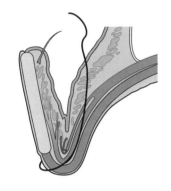

a

b

Figure 4.1

CONGENITAL ECTROPION

AETIOLOGY

True congenital ectropion is usually due to a shortage of skin, an increase in lid length or a combination of both of these.

TREATMENT

1. Maintain the cornea with lubricants and antibiotic ointment as necessary.
2. Consider adding skin as a free graft usually taken from behind the ear.
   Note: Skin grafts in young children are often poor cosmetically and should only be used if necessary for corneal protection.
3. Consider horizontal lid shortening as appropriate.

ACQUIRED ECTROPION

SYSTEM FOR ACQUIRED ECTROPION

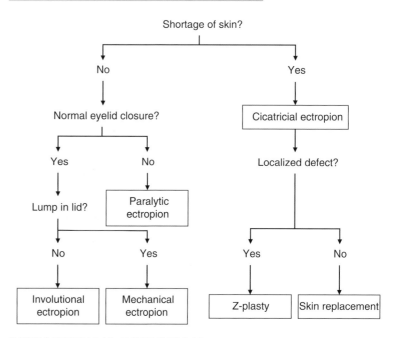

INVOLUTIONAL ECTROPION

PATHOPHYSIOLOGY OF EYELID AGEING CHANGES

Eyelid ageing changes are the same whether they cause ectropion or entropion (see p 32). The fundamental difference between entropion and ectropion is the behaviour of the lamellae when they dissociate. In lower lid entropion the anterior lamella and preseptal muscle moves upwards on the tarsus and posterior lamella whereas in ectropion the anterior lamella is relatively fixed and the posterior lamella moves upwards. When the lid margin begins to evert the tarsus and conjunctiva becomes exposed leading to secondary inflammatory changes and thickening which mechanically increases the ectropion. The main ageing changes which require correction in both involutional ectropion and entropion can be summarised as follows:

- Horizontal lid laxity
- Lower lid retractor weakness
- Lamella dissociation.

AETIOLOGY AND MANAGEMENT OF INVOLUTIONAL ECTROPION

1. **Horizontal lid laxity.** This may be generalised or occur primarily at the lateral or medial canthus. **Treatment.** Tighten the lid in the area of maximum lid laxity.
2. **Lower lid retractor weakness or dissinsertion. Treatment.** Shorten and reattach the lower lid retractors.
3. **Lamella dissociation. Treatment.** Inverting sutures.

See system for lower lid involutional ectropion.

SYSTEM FOR INVOLUTIONAL ECTROPION

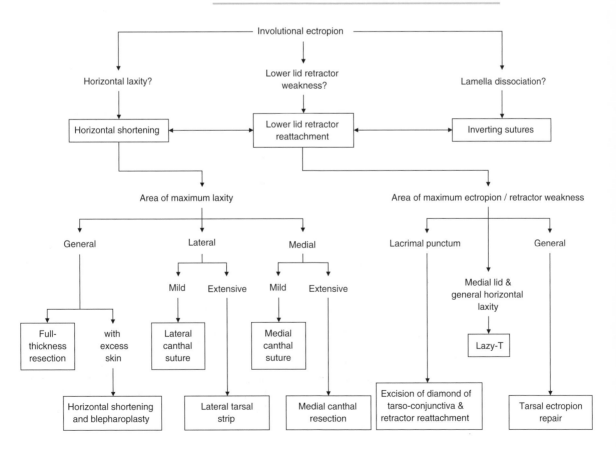

HORIZONTAL LID SHORTENING

Principle
The lid is tightened in area of maximum lid laxity.

Diagnosis
Assess the *site* of maximum laxity by pulling the lid away from the globe and noting where the maximum stretch occurs. Assess the *extent* and significance of the laxity by noting how much the lid can be pulled away from the globe and how quickly the lid reapproximates the globe when it is released (snap test).

Indications
    I. Generalised laxity.
        (a) Full thickness resection of lid.
        (b) With excess skin: horizontal lid shortening and blepharoplasty (Kuhnt-Symanowski procedure)
    II. Lateral canthal laxity.
        (a) Mild/moderate, i.e. laxity in lateral canthal tendon: lateral canthal suture.
        (b) Extensive: lateral tarsal strip.
    III. Medial canthal laxity.
        (a) Mild/moderate: medial canthal suture.
        (b) Extensive: medial canthal resection.

I. GENERALISED LAXITY

A. FULL THICKNESS LID RESECTION (Fig 4.2)

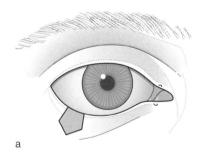

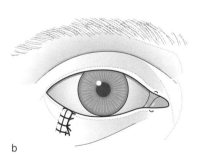

Method
Carry out a pentagonal full thickness lid resection in the area of maximum lid laxity or about 5 mm from the lateral canthus (see Chapter 2).

B. HORIZONTAL LID SHORTENING AND BLEPHAROPLASTY (KUHNT-SYMANOWKSI PROCEDURE) (Fig 4.3)

Principle
Excess skin is excised as a lateral triangle from a blepharoplasty flap and the lid is shortened under the flap.

Indications
Generalised horizontal lid laxity and excess skin.

Figure 4.2

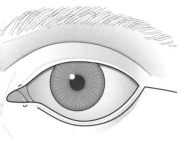
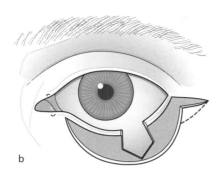
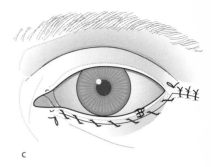

b   c

Figure 4.3

Method

1. Make a subciliary incision 1–2 mm below the lashes from the inferior punctum to the lateral canthus and then follow a skin crease downwards and laterally for about 8 mm (Fig 4.3a).
2. Undermine this skin flap from the orbicularis muscle.
3. Proceed as described for a horizontal lid shortening. Cut through the intact lid margin and remove the rest of the pentagon of lid tissue from under the skin flap (Fig 4.3b).
4. Repair the pentagonal lid defect.
5. Lay the blepharoplasty flap across the reconstructed lid and excise the excess skin as a base-up lateral triangle (Fig 4.3b). Vertical excess skin can be excised as a thin laterally-based triangle (see Fig 12.7d).
6. Suture the subciliary incision with a continuous 6 '0' nylon suture and the lateral skin crease incision with interrupted sutures (Fig 4.3c).

   Note: excess fat can be easily excised if a skin/muscle flap is used instead of a skin flap as described in Chapter 12.

Complications

Shortening of the horizontal palpebral aperture and lower lid retraction. This is usually due to failure to recognise lateral canthal laxity. Treatment: Lateral canthal suture.

II. LATERAL CANTHAL LAXITY

A. **LATERAL CANTHAL SUTURE** (Fig 4.4)

Principle

The lateral tarsus or lateral canthal tendon tissues are sutured to the periosteum of the lateral orbital rim.

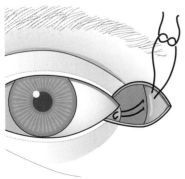

Indications

Mild/moderate lateral canthal tendon laxity.

Figure 4.4

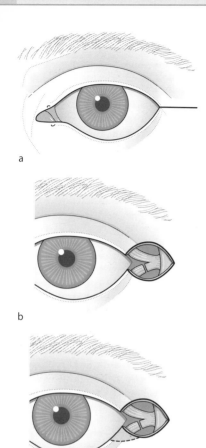

a

b

c

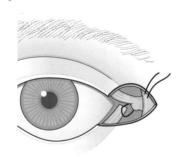

d

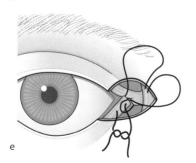

e

Figure 4.5

Method

1. Make a 5 mm skin incision horizontally or rising slightly from the lateral canthus.
2. Deepen the incision and extend it subciliary if necessary for 2–3 mm to allow the lateral canthal tendon, lateral edge of tarsal plate or other tissues to be firmly grasped and approximated to the periosteum of the lateral orbital wall, leaving the lid margin in a normal position against the globe.
3. Pass a suture into the tissue that has been grasped then into the periosteum starting posterior to the orbital rim (Fig 4.4). Tie the suture. Various sutures can be used e.g. 4 or 5 '0' prolene, 5 '0' ethibond or long-acting absorbable sutures. If a double-armed suture is used take a double bite of the grasped tissues and pass each needle through the periosteum and tie the sutures (Fig 4.4).
   Note: If elevation of the lateral canthus is required as well as tightening, a small incision can be made in the lateral upper lid skin crease. This can be deepened to expose the periosteum of the lateral orbital rim above the lateral canthal incision. The sutures can then be passed into the orbital rim periosteum at a higher level than the lateral canthus. It may be necessary to partially free the lateral canthal tendon and tissues below it to allow the lid to be adequately tightened and elevated.
4. Close the orbicularis over the deep suture with a buried 6 '0' long-acting absorbable suture. Close the skin with interrupted sutures.

Complications

Granulomas and inclusion cysts may be caused especially by permanent sutures such as ethibond. Treatment: antibiotics; suture removal.

Recurrence may be due to suture absorption or slippage. Treatment: replace sutures.

Lateral canthal malposition may require suture replacement.

B. LATERAL TARSAL STRIP (Fig 4.5)

Principle

The lid is shortened and a new lateral canthal tendon is created out of the lateral tarsal plate.

Indications

Extensive lateral canthal laxity.

Method

1. Make a horizontal skin incision at the lateral canthus (Fig 4.5a).

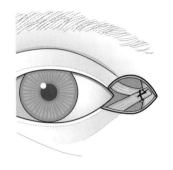

f

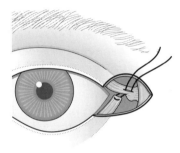

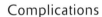

g

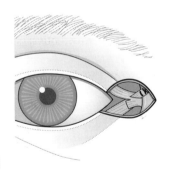

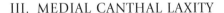

h

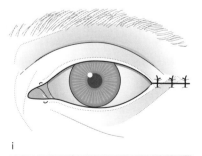

i

Figure 4.5 cont'd

2. Cut the lower limb of the lateral canthal tendon leaving the upper limb intact (Fig 4.5b).

3. Manufacture a new tendon from the lateral part of the tarsal plate by excising skin, orbicularis, lashes and conjunctiva from the tarsus as far as the proposed position of the new lateral canthus which depends on the lid laxity (Fig 4.5c).

4. Expose the periosteum over the lateral orbital rim. Pass each arm of a double-armed suture such as 4/0 prolene into the periosteum starting behind the orbital rim. This leaves a loop of suture under which the strip of tarsus can be pulled (Fig 4.7d). Pass one needle through the tarsal strip just medial to the loop of suture. Pass the other needle through the tarsal strip just lateral to the loop of suture (Fig 4.7e). When the sutures are tightened the loop pulls the tarsal strip posterior to the orbital rim. Tie the sutures together over the loop which fixates it firmly (Fig 4.5f).

   Note: An alternative technique is to pass the lateral tarsal strip through a buttonhole in the upper limb of the lateral canthal tendon to obtain posterior fixation (Fig 4.5g). It can then be sutured directly to the periosteum of the lateral orbital rim to tighten the lid (Fig 4.5h).

5. Close the orbicularis muscle with buried long-acting absorbable sutures and the skin with interrupted sutures (Fig 4.5i).

Complications

Granulomas, inclusion cysts, recurrence and lateral canthal malposition occur as with a lateral canthal suture.

Excess lower lid tightening and reduction of the horizontal palpebral aperture can also occur. This usually resolves with time but if it does not do so the lateral canthus can be opened horizontally with scissors.

III. MEDIAL CANTHAL LAXITY

A. MEDIAL CANTHAL SUTURE

ANTERIOR LIMB STABILISING SUTURE
(Fig 4.6)

Principle

The anterior limb of the medial canthal tendon is stabilised or shortened by suturing the medial end of the lower tarsal plate to the main part of the medial canthal tendon.

Indications

Mild/moderate medial canthal laxity. It is valuable as a stabilising suture when combined with other lid procedures. It is also used to reform the medial canthal tendon in the anophthalmic socket when reformation of the posterior limb of the medial canthal tendon may not be as important as a strong medial canthal reconstruction to support an artificial eye.

Method

1. Make an incision through the skin below the lower canaliculus (Fig 4.6a).
2. Expose the medial end of the tarsal plate.
3. Expose the lower border and insertion of the medial canthal tendon.
4. Pass a 5 '0' nylon or similar non-absorbable suture from the tarsus immediately below the lower punctum to the medial canthal tendon, trying to keep posterior and superior (Fig 4.6b).
5. Tie the suture tight enough to overcome the excess laxity but not so tightly that the inferior canaliculus is bunched up or that the punctum is pulled anteriorly away from the globe (Fig 4.6c).
6. Close the skin incision and remove the skin sutures at 5 days (Fig 4.6d).

Complications

Anteroposition of the lacrimal punctum. If an attempt is made to correct an established malposition of the lacrimal punctum by tightening the anterior limb suture, the punctum will be anteropositioned. A posterior limb reformation is indicated.

POSTERIOR LIMB SUTURE

1. OPEN TECHNIQUE (Fig 4.7)

Principle

The medial orbital wall is exposed allowing the medial canthal tendon reforming sutures to be placed in the periosteum under direct vision. They suture the medial end of the lower tarsal plate to the periosteum over the posterior lacrimal crest (Fig 4.7a). Advantage: accurate placement of sutures. Disadvantage: in older age the periosteum is sometimes not strong enough to hold the sutures adequately.

Indications

Mild/moderate medial canthal laxity in patients with medial ectropion.

Method

1. Make a conjunctival incision through the caruncle and extend it to the medial end of the lower tarsal plate (Fig 4.7b).
2. Put a probe in the inferior canaliculus as a guide and expose the medial orbital wall behind the probe and lacrimal sac using blunt dissection. Clean the periosteum.

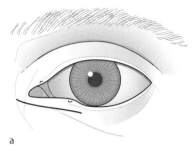

a

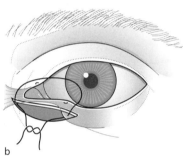

b

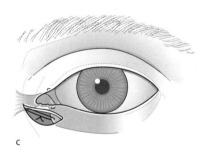

c

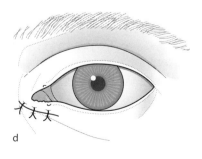

d

Figure 4.6

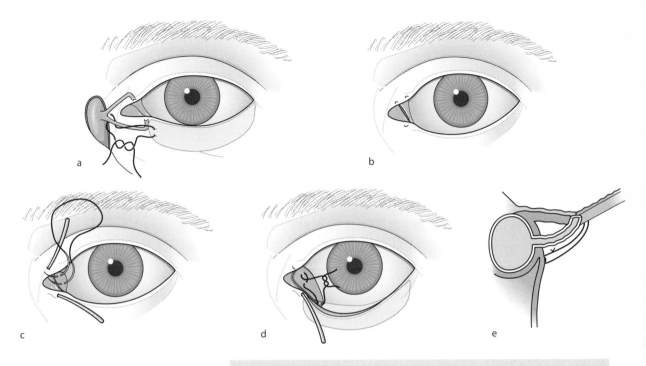

Figure 4.7

3. Take a double armed 5 '0' nonabsorbable suture with half circle needles and pass each needle through the periosteum or firm tissue in the region of the posterior lacrimal crest or a little higher on the medial orbital wall (Fig 4.7c).
4. Pass the needles through the exposed medial end of the tarsus (Fig 4.7d).
5. Position one or more 6 '0' absorbable sutures across the conjunctival wound.
6. Tie the nonabsorbable suture to reform the posterior limb of the medial canthal tendon.
7. Tie the conjunctival suture.

Complications

Exposure of suture. Treatment: remove suture.

Recurrence. Repeat procedure, use closed technique or use mini plate to obtain more secure fixation point.

2. CLOSED TECHNIQUE (Fig 4.8)

Principle

A posterior limb medial canthal tendon reforming stitch is placed without exposing the medial orbital wall.

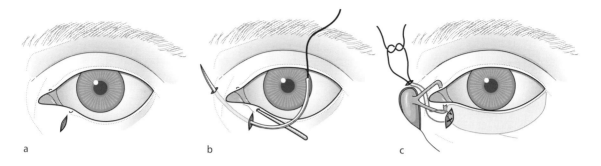

a   b   c

Figure 4.8

Indications

Mild/moderate medial canthal laxity in patients with medial ectropion who require the simplest quickest repair.

Method

1. Make a skin incision below the inferior punctum and expose the medial part of the tarsal plate (Fig 4.8a).
2. Place a probe in the inferior canaliculus.
3. Take a double-armed 4 '0' prolene or similar suture with preferably a 20 mm or larger half circle diameter needle. Pass this twice through the medial end of the tarsal plate as close to the punctum as possible without entering the canaliculus.
4. Hold one of the needles in a large general-purpose needle holder and pass it medially under the canaliculus watching the needle point under the conjunctiva until it reaches the medial canthus. At this point pass the needle posteriorly and engage the medial orbital wall tissue (surgical periosteum) behind and above the fundus of the lacrimal sac. Bring the needle forward to exit through the skin above the medial canthal tendon and below the medial end of the brow (Fig 4.8b).
   Note: if difficulty is experienced passing the needle it is usually because the surgeon is trying to pick up the 'surgical periosteum' too posteriorly.
5. While the needle is still protruding through the skin, make an incision with a no. 11 blade to free the needle down to the periosteum.
6. Pull the needle and suture through the incision.
7. Pass the second needle in a similar way to the first needle and bring it out through the wound created with the no. 11 blade.
8. Tighten the two sutures which should pull the lacrimal punctum medially, posteriorly and upwards (Fig 4.8c).
9. Tie the sutures together and bury the knot deeply within the wound.
10. Close the orbicularis with a buried absorbable suture.
11. Close the skin wounds both below the inferior punctum and the medial canthus with interrupted sutures.

Complications

Recurrence. Treatment: Put in a new suture. If the old suture is not causing any problems simply leave it alone.

B. MEDIAL CANTHAL RESECTION (Fig 4.9)

Principle

Horizontal lid shortening is performed medially. The inferior canaliculus is cut as part of the lid resection and is marsupialised into the conjunctival sac. The posterior limb of the medial canthal tendon is reconstructed.

Indications

Severe medial ectropion with marked laxity of the medial canthal tendon as may occur with long-standing involutional paralytic ectropion.

Method

1. Cut vertically through the full thickness of the lid just lateral to the caruncle. The canaliculus is cut, but try to save as much of it as possible (Fig 4.9a).

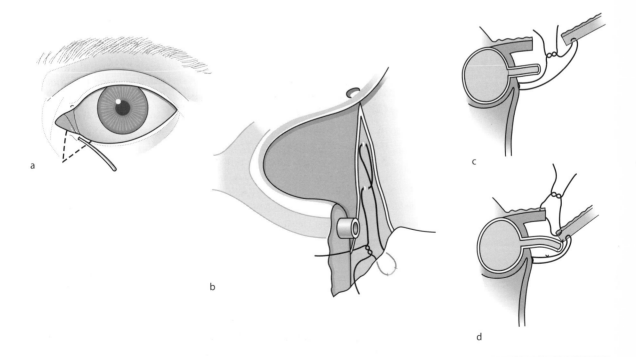

a

b

c

d

Figure 4.9

2. Pass a probe into the cut canaliculus. Palpate the posterior lacrimal crest behind the probe with a blunt-pointed pair of scissors.

3. Spread the scissors and expose the medial orbital wall at or just above the upper end of the posterior lacrimal crest. The exposure is improved if a small malleable retractor is used and the conjunctiva is opened just behind the caruncle, as described for an open reformation of the posterior limb of the medial canthal tendon.

4. Take a 5 '0' double-armed nonabsorbable suture with half-circle needles and pass each needle through the periosteum or firm tissues in the region of the posterior lacrimal crest or just above it on the medial orbital wall (Fig 4.9b).

5. Pull the cut lateral part of the lid towards this fixation suture. Assess how much of the lid needs to be resected and excise this portion.

6. Pass each needle of the fixation suture through the resected tarsus (Fig 4.9c). Before tying it, open the cut canaliculus and suture it to the posterior edge of the tarsus with one or more fine absorbable sutures. Close the conjunctiva with interrupted sutures.

7. Tie the fixation suture to reform the posterior limb of the resected medial canthal tendon and close the skin with 6 '0' interrupted sutures (Fig 4.9d).

Complications

Recurrence. Treatment: Medial canthal suture.
  Granuloma. Treatment: Remove suture.

LOWER LID RETRACTOR SHORTENING/REATTACHMENT

Principle

Shorten and reattach the lower lid retractors to the lower border of the tarsus or the region of the inferior lacrimal punctum.

Diagnosis

Lower lid retractor weakness or dissinsertion is diagnosed by partial or complete ectropion with poor movement of the lid on down gaze. The lacrimal punctum may be ectropic on its own or this may be associated with a general medial horizontal lid laxity. The whole lid may be so everted that it forms a horizontal 'shelf ectropion' which does not correct itself when the patient looks down. The lower lid retractors are totally dissinserted and may be seen as a white area under the conjunctiva in the inferior fornix which moves on down gaze.

A. EXCISION OF DIAMOND OF TARSOCONJUNCTIVA (AND LOWER LID RETRACTOR PLICATION) (Fig 4.10)

Principle

The lower punctum is inverted by vertically shortening the posterior lamella of the lid and tightening the lower lid retractors.

Indications

Lacrimal punctal ectropion with lower lid retractor weakness and without significant horizontal lid laxity.

Method

1. Place a probe in the inferior canaliculus.
2. Excise a diamond of tarsoconjunctiva from below the punctum using a no. 11 blade and scissors. The apex of the diamond should be immediately below the lower punctum, leaving enough space for a suture to enter the tarsus above it without entering the ampulla of the canaliculus (Fig. 4.10a).
3. Make a cut through the conjunctiva from the lateral horizontal apex of the diamond for about 5 mm (Fig 4.10b).

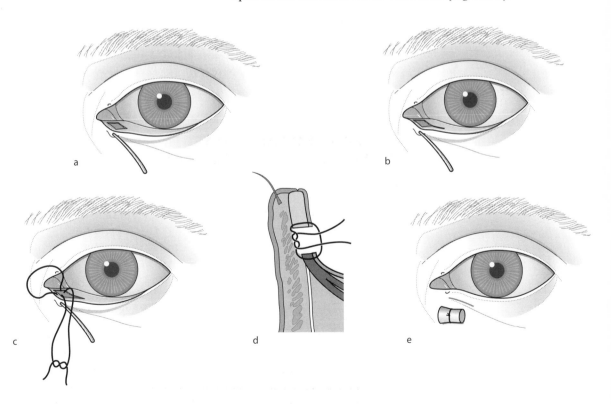

a

b

c

d

e

Figure 4.10

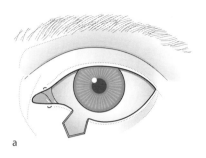

a

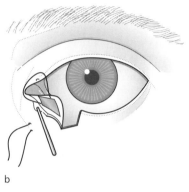

b

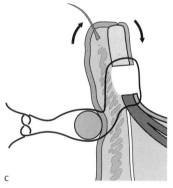

c

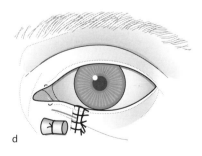

d

Figure 4.11

4. Pass one arm of a double-armed 6 '0' long-acting absorbable suture through the apex of the diamond immediately below the punctum. The lacrimal probe should now be removed. Pass the other arm of the suture through the conjunctiva below the inferior apical cut. Move the suture laterally under the conjunctiva to pick up the lower lid retractors (Fig 4.10c). They are more active in the central than the medial part of the lid. The extension of the conjunctival incision makes picking up the retractors easier.

5. Tie the suture with a knot buried in the wound (Fig 4.10d). It is left to absorb of its own accord and the patient given antibiotic drops and ointment.

Complications

Punctal displacement. If the lower lid retractor shortening suture is displaced too far centrally in the lid the shape of the lid may be distorted. The suture may need to be replaced.

B. LAZY-T (Fig 4.11)

Principle

A full thickness horizontal lid resection is carried out to correct excess horizontal lid laxity. This is coupled with the excision of a diamond of tarsoconjunctiva and a lower lid retractor shortening to invert the lower lacrimal punctum.

Indications

A medial ectropion with horizontal lid laxity which does not predominantly involve the medial canthal tendon.

Method

1. Make an incision through the lid margin about 4 mm lateral to the inferior punctum.
2. Overlap the cut edges and resect a full thickness pentagon of the lid lateral to this first incision (Fig 4.11a).
3. Place a probe in the inferior canaliculus and excise a diamond of tarsoconjunctiva as previously described. Position, but do not tie, a long-acting absorbable suture which picks up the lower lid retractors (Fig 4.10c). Alternatively an inverting suture can be used (Fig 4.11b,c).
4. Repair the horizontal defect and then tie the lower lid retractor shortening suture in the wound (Fig 4.10d) or the inverting suture over a bolster on the skin (Fig 4.11d).
   Note: If each needle of the suture used to shorten the lower lid retractors and close the diamond of tarsoconjunctiva is

brought out through the orbicularis and skin of the eyelid at a lower level than the diamond excision, it will act both to shorten the lower lid retractors and as an inverting suture.

Complications

Eyelid margin notch. If the medial fragment of the eyelid is inverted too aggressively a notch may occur. Treatment: Revision of wound.

C. TARSAL ECTROPION REPAIR (TARSAL EVERSION OR SHELF ECTROPION) (Fig 4.12)

Principle

The lower lid retractors are reattached to the lower border of the tarsus usually via a posterior conjunctival approach.

Indications

Partial or total lower lid retractor disinsertion. The lower lid retractors can be shortened and reattached to the lower border of the tarsus. This is often associated with other inverting procedures.

Method

1. Place a lower lid traction suture through the grey-line (Fig 4.12a).
2. Make an incision through the conjunctiva just below the tarsal plate (Fig 4.12b).
3. Undermine the conjunctiva to the lower lid retractors. Identify them by getting the patient to look up and down. See and feel them move.

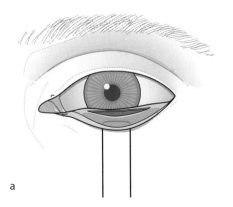
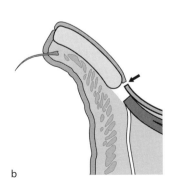
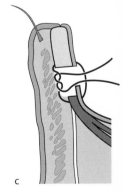

a   b   c

Figure 4.12

4. Pass a long-acting absorbable suture through the lower lid retractors, through the inferior cut edge of the conjunctiva, through the lower border of the tarsal plate and tie it with a bow knot in the wound. If this produces lid retraction replace the suture taking a smaller bite of the retractors. If it does not invert the lid take a deeper bite of the retractors (Fig 4.12c).

5. When the suture placement is satisfactory, place two more sutures on either side of the midline suture and tie them with the knots within the wound and away from the cornea.

6. Remove traction suture.

Complications

Inadequate inversion. Treatment: Consider tightening lid and adding inverting sutures.

LAMELLA DISSOCIATION

INVERTING SUTURES (Fig 4.13)

Principle

A double-armed suture is passed from the conjunctiva just below the inferior tarsus through the orbicularis and is tied on the skin at a lower level (Fig 4.13a,b). In the upper lid the suture is passed from just above the upper tarsus and tied on the skin at a much higher level (see acute eversion – Fig 4.1) This inverts the lid, corrects the lamella dissociation, binds the lamellae together and repositions them.

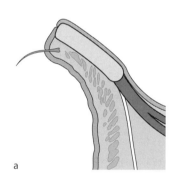

a

Indications

To correct ectropion caused by lamella disassociation which may occur with any cause of conjunctival oedema, e.g. acute eversion, severe blepharoconjunctivitis, allergic reactions etc. Inverting sutures can be used to help inversion in many ectropion procedures.

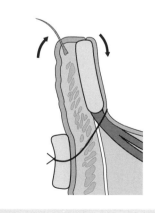

b

Figure 4.13

Method

1. Pass each needle of a 4/0 long-acting absorbable suture from the conjunctiva just below the lower border of the tarsus and come out through the orbicularis and skin at a lower level (Fig 4.13). Do the reverse with the upper lid (see Fig 4.1).

2. Tighten the sutures sufficiently and tie them over a bolster so that the lid margin is inverted a little more than is required. Remove the sutures after about 1–2 weeks or as appropriate i.e. when the lid swelling has subsided etc.

MECHANICAL ECTROPION (Fig 4.14)

AETIOLOGY

Tumours or cysts near the lid margin can mechanically cause an ectropion.

TREATMENT

Excise the cause. The lesion should be excised as vertically as possible to prevent a cicatricial ectropion (Fig. 4.14a). If the lesion is associated with horizontal lid laxity the lid should be shortened at the same time (Fig 4.14b).

CICATRICIAL ECTROPION

AETIOLOGY

The lid margin is pulled away from the globe by a shortage of skin, which can be due to a variety of causes, e.g. congenital shortage, trauma, burns, skin conditions, cicatrising skin tumours, medications, allergies, actinic and general involutional changes leading to a loss of skin elasticity often aggravated by cheek ptosis. Both eyelids may be involved and the shortage of skin may be local or general.

Diagnosis

If in doubt about the diagnosis on the appearance alone, push the lower lid up or the upper lid down over the eyeball with a finger. If the lid cannot be stretched in this way there is shortage of skin causing the cicatricial ectropion.

Indications

Local linear shortage of skin: Z-plasty.
General shortage of skin: skin graft or flap.

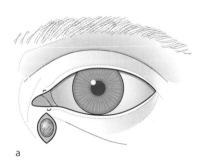

a

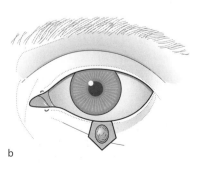

b

Figure 4.14

Z-PLASTY (Fig 4.15)

Principle

Two flaps of skin are transposed (Fig 4.15a). This:
- increases the length of skin in the line of the scar contraction at the expense of shortening the skin at right angles to it;
- alters the line of the scar.

Indications

To lengthen a localised scar, e.g. cicatricial ectropion, or to improve the appearance of a scar by breaking up its continuity.

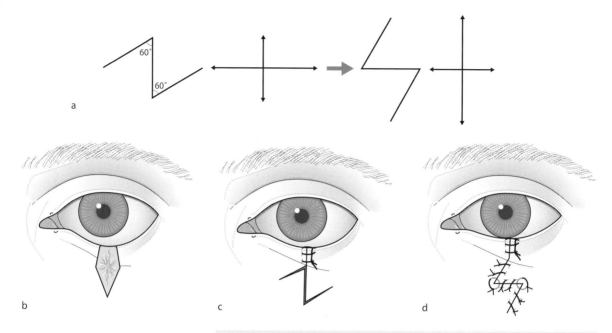

Figure 4.15

Method

1. If the lid margin is involved in the scar, excise the notch first and repair this defect before planning the Z-plasty (Fig 4.15b,c).
2. Mark the line of the scar. From each end mark another line the same length as the scar line but running at 60° to it, making a 'Z' shape (Fig 4.15c). If the scar is long it is better to make more than one Z, keeping the limbs all the same length (p 163).
3. Cut the skin flaps and excise the deep scar tissue.
4. Transpose and suture the flaps (Fig 4.15d).
5. Put a 4 '0' traction suture through the lid margin in the line of the original scar (or place two traction sutures, one on each side of a lid margin repair) and keep the lid on traction for 48 hours postoperatively.

Complications

Inadequate vertical lengthening of the scar and correction of the ectropion may be related to insufficient horizontal laxity. Treatment: mobilise or add tissue, e.g. as a graft or flap.

Scarring of flaps. Treatment: massage, local steroids.

SKIN REPLACEMENT (Fig 4.16)

Principle

Skin can be replaced with a flap or graft. A local flap is preferable if one is available. If a graft is used, suitably thinned full-thickness skin is

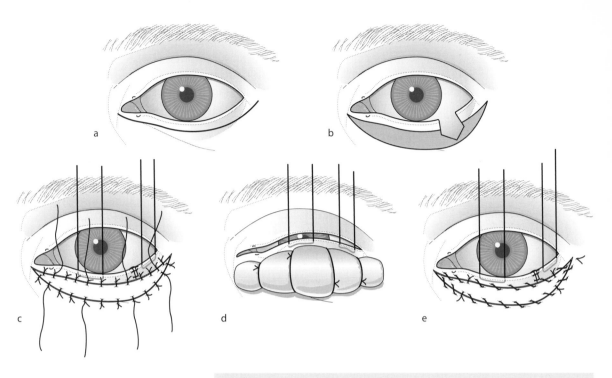

Figure 4.16

preferable to split-thickness skin for both the upper and lower lids unless the defect is too large, there is not enough full-thickness skin available, e.g. in burns, or the graft bed is suspect. A graft must be held against its bed with either fixation sutures, a bolster or a simple pressure dressing. The viability of flaps used in eyelid reconstruction is often dependent on the take of part of the flap as a free graft. A pressure dressing or fixation is therefore often desirable for flaps as well as for grafts, in contrast to the principles of reconstruction elsewhere.

Indications

A generalised shortage of skin.

Method

1. Create the defect, i.e. make an incision approximately parallel to the lid margin through the area of shortage and free the skin and scar tissue until the ectropion is corrected (Fig 4.16a).
2. Carry out a horizontal lid resection if there is excess lid laxity, which is usually the case if the ectropion has been present for a long time (Fig 4.16b).
3. Place two lid traction sutures in the lid margin to exaggerate the defect.

4. Cut a local flap or graft as required (p 12). Close the donor site. Suture the skin into the defect. Classically a skin graft is held against its bed with sutures tied over a bolster (Fig 4.16c,d). This tends to evert the lid margin and perpetuate the ectropion. It is preferable to suture the graft with a fine continuous absorbable suture and to apply a local pressure dressing for 48 hours without tie-over sutures (Fig 4.16e).

   Note: if the graft is large and there is a risk of haemorrhage under it, make stab incisions in it so that any blood can be absorbed into the overlying pressure dressing.

5. Keep the lid on traction for 48 hours postoperatively.

   Note: a. A local medial or lateral transposition flap from the upper lid is useful for small degrees of cicatricial ectropion.

   b. A free skin graft should, where possible, be extended beyond the horizontal limits of the canthi so that when the graft contracts there is some theoretical medial and lateral support for the lid.

   c. If cheek ptosis is significant, its correction often with lateral canthal support can significantly improve lid retraction and cicatricial ectropion. This may reduce or obviate the need for skin grafting.

Complications

Haemorrhage under the graft. Treatment: if haematoma is fluctuant, aspirate it with a syringe and wide-bore needle; give systemic antibiotics; reapply pressure dressing.

Insufficient correction. Treatment: if mild this can sometimes be improved with a lid tightening procedure or lateral canthal support and elevation. If more severe, add more tissue or raise cheek.

PARALYTIC ECTROPION

Aetiology

7th nerve palsy. The paralysed orbicularis muscle stretches. This is usually most obvious where the muscle becomes continuous with the medial and lateral canthal tendons. Correction requires support for the paralysed lid and tightening to correct the lid laxity. If the 7th nerve palsy and paralytic ectropion is long-standing, secondary changes of skin contraction and cheek ptosis may occur.

Diagnosis

Inability to close eyelids fully in absence of skin shortage or scarring.

Management.

1. Support
   a. Medial:
      – Lee medial canthoplasty

- medial tarsorrhaphy
   b. Lateral:
      – lateral canthal elevation
      – lateral tarsorrhaphy
   c. General:
      – fascial sling
2. Tighten
   a. Medial:
      – medial canthal suture
      – medial canthal resection
   b. Lateral:
      – lateral canthal suture
      – lateral tarsal strip
3. Correction of secondary changes to support lid:
      – skin graft
      – cheek/mid face lift.

SYSTEM FOR PARALYTIC LOWER LID ECTROPION

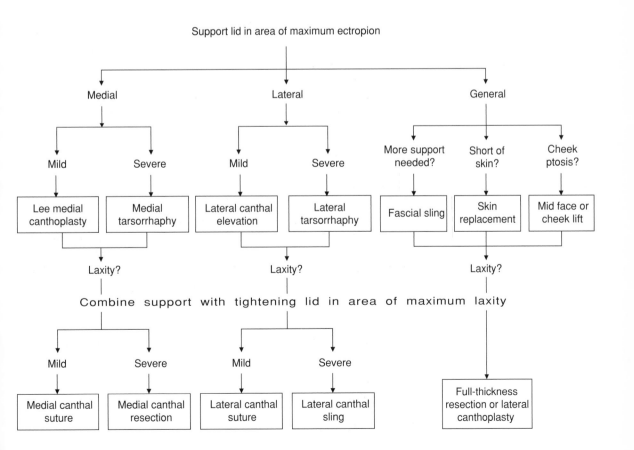

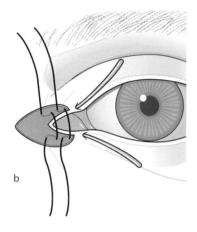

a

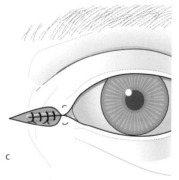

b

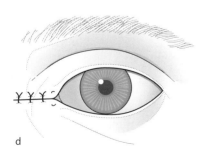

c

d

Figure 4.17

LEE MEDIAL CANTHOPLASTY (Fig 4.17)

Principle

The eyelids are sutured together medial to the lacrimal puncta to support the lower lid and reduce the increased vertical interpalpebral distance at the medial canthus and to bring the lacrimal puncta into the tearfilm.

Indications

Mild paralytic medial ectropion without marked medial canthal tendon laxity; an increased vertical interpalpebral distance associated with lid retraction, trauma, etc.

Method

1. Pass a probe into each canaliculus.
2. Split both the lid margins medial to the puncta and anterior to the probes with a small no. 11 blade (Fig 4.17a).
3. Undermine the skin for about 5 mm.
4. Take a deep horizontal bite with a 6 '0' long-acting absorbable suture passed into the orbicularis muscle below the inferior canaliculus and above the superior canaliculus. A second suture may be added depending on the extent of the tarsorrhaphy desired (Fig 4.17b). When the sutures are tied the two canaliculae are approximated, the lower lid elevated, and the puncta inverted (Fig 4.17c).
5. Suture the skin edges after excising any excess skin if necessary (Fig 4.17d).

Complications

Damage to the canaliculae
    Alteration of the normal medial canthal angle.

MEDIAL TARSORRHAPHY (Fig 4.18)

Principle

A 'central' tarsorrhaphy is carried out just lateral to the lacrimal puncta. It supports the medial part of the lower lid and protects the cornea. It can be reversed at any time.

Indications

Acute 7th nerve palsy as temporary measure for corneal protection and control of the paralytic ectropion. It is rarely required for established paralytic ectropion because of poor cosmesis.

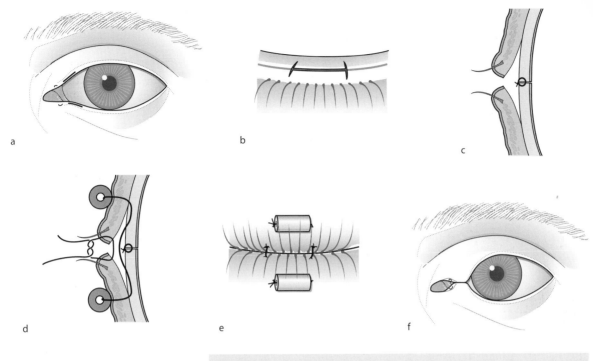

Figure 4.18

Method

1. Make an incision the length of the required tarsorrhaphy through the grey-line of both eyelids using a no. 11 blade (this is usually about 4 mm) (Fig 4.18a).
2. At each end of this incision make a very small cut at right angles to the lid margin but not through its extremities. This makes the wound H-shaped (Fig 4.18b).
3. Evert each split lid margin and suture the raw surfaces of the two tarsal plates together with a buried 6 '0' long-acting absorbable suture. This must not extend through the full thickness of the tarsal plates or it may abrade the cornea (Fig 4.18c).
4. Pass a mattress suture through the centre of the wound and tie it over bolsters on the skin of the upper and lower lids.
5. Suture the everted anterior lamellae together with a skin suture to complete the three-layer closure (Fig 4.18d,e).
6. Remove the mattress suture at 2–3 weeks (Fig 4.18f).

   Note: this type of tarsorrhaphy can be done anywhere along the lid margin, and can be left as a permanent tarsorrhaphy although the interpalpebral junction will tend to stretch.

Complications

Stretching. If the medial tarsorrhaphy is very small and left for a long time the lids will tend to distract stretching the bridge.

Trichiasis. This can occur when the bridge is divided but is rare since no tissue has been excised.

LATERAL CANTHAL ELEVATION (Fig 4.19)

Principle

The lateral canthus can be supported with a lateral canthal suture. Division of the lateral canthal tendon and associated structures may be required to allow the canthus to be elevated sufficiently. A shortage of lower lid skin can be corrected with the transposition of a pedicle flap of skin from the upper to the lower lid. This allows good exposure for the lateral canthal surgery.

Indications

Lateral canthal depression e.g. 7th nerve palsy, trauma, mild cicatricial changes etc. N.B. If a patient complains of epiphora from the lateral canthus they require lateral canthal surgery.

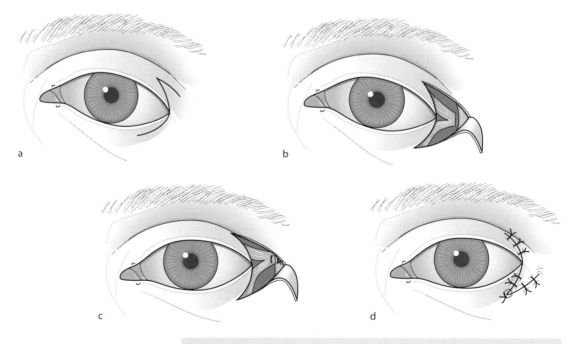

a   b

c   d

Figure 4.19

Method

1. Raise a skin and muscle pedicle flap from the upper lid with the base immediately above the lateral canthus and wide enough to elevate the lateral canthus by the amount required.
2. Make a subciliary skin and muscle incision in the lower lid from the lateral canthus of the same length as the upper lid pedicle flap (Fig 4.19a).
3. Cut the lateral canthal tendon and anything else, e.g. orbital septum, which prevents the lateral canthus from being elevated to the desired level (Fig 4.19b).
4. Suture the lateral canthus directly to the periosteum of the lateral orbital wall at the desired level (Fig 4.19c).
5. Transpose the pedicle flap and suture it into position with interrupted sutures (Fig 4.19d).

   Note: a. If the lateral canthal tendon is lax and there is enough skin below the lateral canthus, a lateral suture may be sufficient on its own to elevate, support and tighten the lid.

   b. The support and corneal protection can be increased if a lateral tarsorrhaphy is combined with the lateral canthal elevation.

Complications

A small pedicle transposition flap may take a long time to settle and give a cosmetically acceptable colour match and contour.

The canthus may be positioned cosmetically and functionally either too high or too low.

LATERAL TARSORRHAPY (See Figs 9.1 and 9.4)

Principle

The lateral eyelids are sutured together either as a 'temporary' or 'permanent' tarsorrhaphy (p 178 and 183). This supports the lower lid and increases corneal protection.

Indications

Corneal exposure from any cause, increased horizontal palpebral aperture and lower lid depression when the upper lid is retracted, e.g. 7th nerve palsy, proptosis etc. A lateral tarsorrhaphy can be combined with a lateral canthal elevation and/or a lateral tarsal strip.

Method

See p 178 and 183.

FASCIAL SLING (See Fig 11.10)

Principle

A strip of fascia is passed through the lid from the medial canthal tendon to the lateral orbital wall.

Indications

Support for the lower lid where medial and lateral canthal surgery is insufficient, e.g. recurrent paralytic ectropion, heavy artificial eye etc.

Method

See p 219.

TIGHTEN LID (SEE INVOLUTIONAL ECTROPION)

Horizontal lid laxity: horizontal lid shortening in area of maximum laxity.

CORRECTION OF SECONDARY CHANGES

Diagnosis

If it is not possible to correct a paralytic lower lid ectropion by gently repositioning the lower lid with a finger, secondary changes of either a cheek ptosis or skin contraction may be present. If pushing up the cheek allows the ectropion to be gently repositioned with a finger, consider carrying out a cheek lift usually with additional canthal surgery. If pushing up the cheek does not allow the ectropion to be manually corrected because of skin changes, carry out a skin graft again usually with canthal surgery.

SKIN GRAFT

Principle

If the 7th nerve palsy is long-standing, secondary changes of skin contraction can occur which increase the paralytic ectropion and lid retraction. These may require skin grafting. See cicatricial ectropion (p 73).

CHEEK PTOSIS

Principle

In cases of long-standing 7th nerve palsy the weight of the paralysed cheek leads to a cheek ptosis. This may require correction with a cheek or mid face lift. See cheek lift (p 248).

Ptosis

5

ASSESSMENT

- Classification
- History
- Examination

CLASSIFICATION OF PTOSIS

- Dysgenetic
- Aponeurotic
- Neurogenic
- Myogenic
- Myasthenic
- Mechanical
- Pseudo ptosis

If a patient is born with ptosis it is by definition congenital. The majority of such cases are due to dysgeneses or malformation of the levator muscle. A child can also be born with a ptosis due to other causes such as aponeurotic defects, nerve palsies etc. Since these can also be acquired after birth, ptosis management will be considered separately for each cause.

HISTORY

The purpose of taking a history is to suggest the provisional diagnosis of the ptosis. In addition to the ophthalmic and general medical history, salient questions should include:

- Duration, e.g. was the patient born with it or was it acquired and if so when did they first notice it.
- Predisposing factors, e.g. history of the pregnancy and delivery, trauma, medical conditions etc.
- Associated symptoms, e.g. jaw-winking, diplopia, dysphagia, tiredness
- Variability, e.g. time of day, progression

- Family history, e.g. some forms of congenital and hereditary ptosis, blepharophimosis, ocular myopathies.

EXAMINATION

The purpose of the examination is to confirm the provisional diagnosis and decide on treatment. In addition to a full ocular examination the following must be noted:

- Presence and degree of ptosis
- Levator function
- Lid position on downgaze
- Skin crease
- Bell's phenomenon
- Associated signs.

PRESENCE AND DEGREE OF PTOSIS

1. Compare lid levels. The upper lid normally covers the limbus by 1–2 mm. This differentiates a unilateral ptosis from contralateral lid retraction. Note any frontalis overaction which may mask a bilateral ptosis.
2. Measure the difference between the corneal light reflex and the upper lid margin when each eye fixes a spot source of light. This is known as the margin reflex distance or MRD. Note any vertical squint or pseudo ptosis.
3. Measure the vertical interpalpebral distances. If the difference is not the same as the MRD difference, it suggests lower lid asymmetry.

LEVATOR FUNCTION

Having established the presence of a true ptosis, the treatment depends mainly on the levator function. Measure the maximum excursion of the lid between full upgaze and downgaze with the frontalis muscle prevented from acting by pressure over the brow (normal 15–18 mm).

LID POSITION ON DOWNGAZE

Lid lag on downgaze in the absence of previous surgery, trauma, etc., suggests a dysgenesis of the levator muscle since the dysgenetic muscle will neither relax nor contract properly. This helps to differentiate the common unilateral congenital dysgenetic ptosis from other causes.

SKIN CREASE

The height of the skin crease should be measured for symmetry at operation and for diagnosis. A high skin crease suggests an aponeurotic defect. The depth of the crease is a guide to the probable levator function in a child who is too young to cooperate. The important measurement for symmetry is the 'upper lid show' or amount of eyelid which is visible between the eyelashes and the edge of the overhanging fold of upper lid skin (see Chapter 1). This depends on the position of the skin crease, the height of the eyelid and the amount of skin in the upper lid.

BELL'S PHENOMENON

If the eye does not rotate upwards on lid closure there is a risk of postoperative corneal exposure, which will affect the choice and extent of any ptosis operation.

ASSOCIATED SIGNS

The following must be specifically looked for:
- Aberrant eyelid movements, e.g. jaw-winking, aberrant third nerve regeneration syndromes
- Pupillary changes, e.g. Horner's syndrome, third nerve palsy
- Fundus abnormality, e.g. pigmentary retinopathy in some ophthalmoplegias
- Myasthenic signs, e.g. fatigueability, hypometric saccades, Cogan twitch.

MANAGEMENT

DYSGENETIC PTOSIS

- Congenital dysgenetic ptosis
- With superior rectus weakness
- Blepharophimosis.

CONGENITAL DYSGENETIC PTOSIS

PATHOPHYSIOLOGY

The levator muscle is dysgenetic and made up of varying proportions of striated muscle fibres with fat and fibrous tissue. The cause of the dysgenesis is probably multifactorial and a combination of genetic and environmental factors. The ptosis is often unilateral but can be bilateral. The less striated muscle and the more fat and fibrous tissue present, the greater degree of ptosis and the worse the levator function. Fibrous tissue is not elastic. Therefore there will be lid lag on downgaze which will increase the more the dysgenetic muscle is shortened to correct the ptosis. If there is less than about 4 mm of levator function the levator muscle will usually be too dysgenetic to support the lid without causing excessive lid lag and there is a significant chance that the dysgenetic muscle will stretch with time causing the ptosis to recur. An alternative source of power must be found to raise the lid and this is usually the frontalis muscle.

TIMING OF SURGERY

The surgery should be performed whenever accurate measurements can be obtained. This is usually when the child is between 3 and 4 years of age prior to proper school. If there is a risk of amblyopia because of the severity of the ptosis, it is justifiable to carry out a brow suspension/frontalis sling procedure at any age using nonautogenous material. There is increasing evidence to show that even if a ptosis only partially occludes the pupil there is a risk of amblyopia and ptosis surgery should be carried out as soon as possible in such cases.

CHOICE OF OPERATION

The choice of operation depends primarily on the levator function as on the system. A severe unilateral ptosis presents the surgeon with a difficult choice between a very large levator resection, if necessary suturing Whitnall's superior suspensory ligament to the tarsus to act as an internal sling (p 102, stage 9), or a brow suspension procedure (p 108). A large levator resection is a unilateral procedure, but if the levator muscle is very dysgenetic it will stretch and the ptosis will recur. If Whitnall's ligament has been sutured to the tarsus the ptosis will not recur, but there will be marked lagophthalmos and asymmetry on downgaze. A brow suspension/frontalis sling can give a more symmetrical result if the procedure is bilateral and if the normal levator muscle is weakened to make both eyelids dependent on the frontalis muscle for elevation. Many parents and patients, however, are unwilling to accept a bilateral procedure for a unilateral condition.

DYSGENETIC PTOSIS WITH SUPERIOR RECTUS WEAKNESS

If the eye is straight in the primary position of gaze but the superior rectus muscle is weak, more extensive ptosis surgery is required to lift the lid by a given amount since the superior rectus muscle normally contributes to upper lid movement via its common sheath with the levator muscle. When a levator resection is performed, an extra 4 mm of levator muscle is arbitrarily resected. If the eye is hypotropic in the primary position, it must be elevated before the ptosis is corrected (see p 92).

BLEPHAROPHIMOSIS

The condition comprises bilateral dysgenetic ptosis, blepharophimosis, telecanthus and epicanthus inversus. There is frequently an

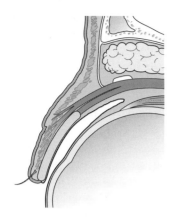

Figure 5.1

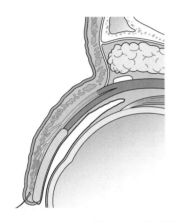

Figure 5.2

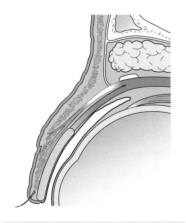

Figure 5.3

associated lower lid ectropion. It is inherited as an autosomal dominant but many sporadic cases occur. The syndrome may occur as part of other conditions. Treatment of the ptosis depends on the levator function. This is usually poor and a bilateral brow suspension/frontalis sling procedure is required when the child's leg is large enough to obtain autogenous fascia lata. As previously stated under simple congenital dysgenetic ptosis, if there is a risk of amblyopia because of the severity of the ptosis it is justifiable to carry out a brow suspension/frontalis sling procedure at any age using nonautogenous material. The epicanthus and telecanthus should be corrected six months prior to the definitive ptosis surgery (p 154).

APONEUROTIC DEFECTS (Figs 5.1, 5.2 and 5.3)

- Congenital
- Acquired: involutional, trauma, oedema, blepharochalasis, etc.

The usual features of an aponeurotic defect are a ptosis which is constant in all positions of gaze, good levator function, a raised skin crease, deep upper lid sulcus and a thinned lid which can be almost transparent. This is caused by a generalised weakness or dissinsertion of the aponeurosis (Fig 5.2) and is analogous to the weakness of the lower lid retractors, which causes involutional entropion. It can be termed a low aponeurotic defect to distinguish it from the less common high aponeurotic defect in which there is fatty change at the musculo-aponeurotic junction (Fig 5.3). These patients have a ptosis that is constant in all positions of gaze. They usually have good levator function but the skin crease is normal and the lid is not thinned. Both types of defect may be congenital or acquired. The ptosis often gets worse at the end of the day, simulating myasthenia. This is because the lid is elevated by Müller's muscle, which fatigues. Aponeurotic defects can be repaired either by an anterior or a posterior approach, preferably under local anaesthesia except in the very young.

NEUROGENIC DEFECTS

- Third nerve and associated syndromes
- Horner's syndrome.

THIRD NERVE PALSY

This varies in degree. If Bell's phenomenon is absent the palsy is difficult to treat surgically. The squint should be corrected first with horizontal muscle surgery and if necessary the superior oblique muscle can be transposed adjacent to the insertion of the medial rectus to hold the eye slightly in adduction. The ptosis should then be corrected depending on the levator function and Bell's phenomenon. If the palsy is total and surgery must be undertaken, a brow suspension can be considered, but the lids must be set low enough to allow complete lid closure when the frontalis muscle is relaxed. If the orbicularis muscle is working normally these patients often benefit from the elasticity of a silicone rod used for the brow suspension.

ABERRANT THIRD NERVE REGENERATION SYNDROMES

The aberrant movement of an eyelid can be abolished by excising the levator muscle and correcting the ptosis with a brow suspension, but there will be a risk of corneal exposure if Bell's phenomenon is poor or absent.

MARCUS GUNN JAW-WINKING PTOSIS

If the ptosis is the main problem it can be corrected by ptosis surgery based on the levator function. If the aberrant movement of the eyelid is the main problem it can be corrected by a levator division or excision and brow suspension procedure. This can be done bilaterally to obtain the most symmetrical result.

HORNER'S SYNDROME

This usually does well with a Fasanella Servat procedure.

MYOGENIC PTOSIS

External ophthalmoplegia and the ocular myopathies are progressive. They involve the extraocular and levator muscles and may progress to involve the frontalis and orbicularis muscles. Ptosis surgery can be undertaken based on the:

- Levator function
- Frontalis action
- Orbicularis power.

The patient must accept that whatever surgical procedure is carried out, further procedures are likely to be required as the condition progresses. Ptosis props are not usually well tolerated initially unless the orbicularis power is significantly reduced.

   If the levator function is more than about 7 mm a levator advancement should be carried out. If the condition progresses and the patient starts to get corneal exposure problems due to a combination of limited eyelid closure and a poor Bell's phenomenon, an upper lid retractor recession may become necessary. If the subsequent ptosis requires correction and the frontalis muscle is working well, e.g. resulting in 5–10+ mm of brow movement, a brow

SYSTEM FOR MYOGENIC PTOSIS

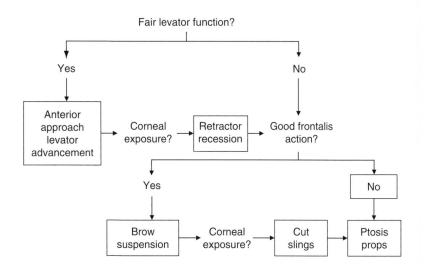

suspension/frontalis sling can be performed, preferably using nonautogenous material under local anaesthesia. In younger patients autogenous fascia lata can be used under general anaesthesia. The eyelids should be left just closed at the end of the operation and if the surgery is performed under general anaesthesia, a careful watch should be kept on the heart. If the condition progresses after a frontalis sling and the patient develops corneal exposure, the lids must be lowered until there is complete eyelid closure at rest. By this stage the orbicularis power is so weak that the patient will usually tolerate ptosis props.

MYASTHENIA

The variability of the condition and possibility of diplopia make ptosis props usually preferable to surgery unless the condition has been stable for a long time.

MECHANICAL PTOSIS

- Eyelid tumours
- Cicatricial conditions
- Trauma.

Eyelid tumours require excision, cicatricial conditions may respond to grafting, and traumatic ptosis usually requires an exploration of the lid, preferably under local anaesthesia.

PSEUDOPTOSIS

This includes all conditions that may simulate a true ptosis, and the treatment depends on the condition e.g.

- Enophthalmos: prosthesis, volume replacement
- Dermatochalasis: blepharoplasty
- Hypotropia and pseudoptosis: Knapp procedure.

PSEUDOPTOSIS AND HYPOTROPIA

If the eye is hypotropic in the primary position, it must be elevated before the ptosis correction. A forced duction test is carried out first and if this shows restriction of elevation, the inferior rectus muscle is freed and recessed if necessary. The horizontal rectus muscle insertions are then moved up adjacent to the insertion of the superior rectus, as described by Knapp. The muscles can be recessed or resected at the same time to improve any horizontal ocular deviation. When there is concern about anterior segment ischaemia, e.g. with patients aged over 25 years old, it is not necessary to disinsert the three rectus muscles at the same time. The inferior rectus muscle is recessed but the horizontal and superior rectus muscle bellies are split longitudinally and sutured to the sclera with a nonabsorbable suture, as suggested by Callahan.

SYSTEM FOR PSEUDOPTOSIS AND HYPOTROPIA

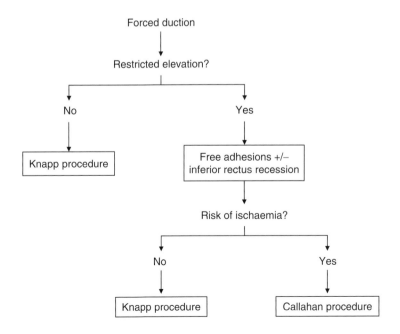

PTOSIS SURGERY

ANAESTHESIA

Local anaesthesia is preferable to general anaesthesia if the patient will tolerate it since the voluntary movement of the levator muscle aids in the identification of lid structures and a better operative assessment of lid level is possible.

Method

1. Mark the skin crease.
2. Evert the lid and inject 1 or 2 ml of local anaesthetic immediately under the conjunctiva just above the upper border of the tarsal plate.
3. Give a subcutaneous injection in the region of the skin crease.
   Note: a. Epinephrine in the local anaesthetic helps to reduce bleeding but stimulates Müller's muscle.
   b. A frontal nerve block is not usually necessary and runs a risk of affecting the function of the levator muscle.
   c. The addition of a long-acting anaesthetic such as bupivacaine (Marcain) greatly prolongs the time available for surgery and postpones the need for further injections during the operation which distort tissues, etc.

SYSTEM FOR PTOSIS SURGERY

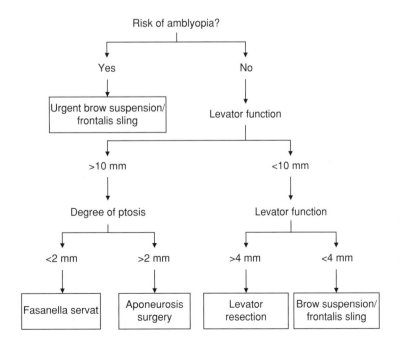

FASANELLA SERVAT PROCEDURE (Fig 5.4)

Principle

The upper border of tarsus is excised with the lower part of Müller's muscle and the overlying conjunctiva (Fig 5.4a).

Indications

Mild congenital ptosis with a levator function better than 10 mm; Horner's syndrome; small degrees of involutional ptosis if not associated with a frank aponeurotic weakness; minor contour adjustment after previous ptosis or other upper lid surgery.

Method

1. Make a stab incision through the skin crease in the most lateral part of the lid.
2. Evert the lid and clamp two curved micro-artery forceps over the upper attached border of the tarsus and lower part of Müller's muscle with its overlying conjunctiva.

   Note: a. the curved artery forceps should be applied as in Figure 5.4b to compensate for the tendency to excise excess tissue from the centre of the lid due to the curve of the upper attached border of the tarsal plate. This can cause central peaking of the lid.

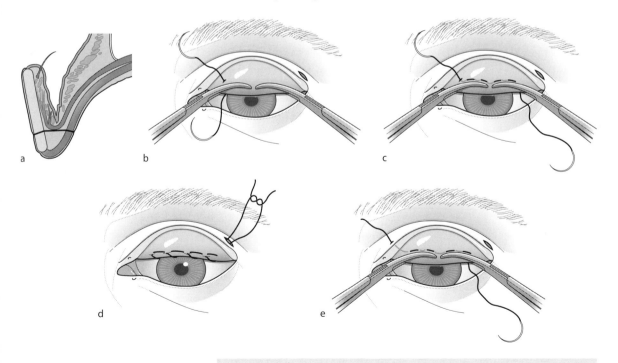

a   b   c

d   e

Figure 5.4

    b. a small adjustment in the amount resected and there-fore the elevation and contour achieved is possible by altering the position of the artery forceps and by pulling more tarsus, conjunctiva and Muller's muscle through them using fine-toothed forceps.

3. Pass one needle of a double-armed 6 '0' absorbable suture through the everted lid immediately below the artery forceps (Fig 5.4b). Start medially and continue laterally as a running suture through the lid, taking about four to six bites (Fig 5.4c).

4. Remove the artery forceps and cut along the crush marks with scissors.

5. Use the other arm of the absorbable suture to approximate the cut edges of the wound. Stay superficial and take care not to cut the first suture with the passage of the second needle.

6. Pass both arms of the suture through the conjunctival wound in the lateral part of the lid and out through the stab incision in the skin. Tie them without tension and bury the knot beneath the skin which does not need to be sutured (Fig 5.4d).

    Note: a. An initial postoperative lateral droop of the lid is usual. This corrects itself as the suture knot absorbs.

        b. An alternative technique is to pass a 5 '0' nylon suture through the lid medially leaving one end of the suture on the skin. Run the suture below the artery forceps instead of the absorbable suture – stage 3 (Fig 5.4e). Bring it out laterally through the lid after cutting along the crush marks – stage 4. Tape the ends of the suture to the skin and remove it after about 5 days. This suture can be easily and completely removed at any time, e.g. to prevent corneal irritation, but the correction obtained is less than with the other method. The suture may be pulled out inadvertently and hence this technique is better reserved for adults.

Complications

Corneal abrasion; foreign body sensation; central peaking; difficulty with subsequent upper lid surgery due to reduction of tarsus; skin crease lowering: this will happen if the height of the tarsal plate is reduced below the preoperative skin crease level.

APONEUROSIS SURGERY

Aponeurosis surgery is indicated for patients with an aponeurotic defect and good levator function, i.e. usually better than 10 mm. Local anaesthesia should be used if at all possible and the lid set at operation to the same level or a little higher than the other side. Aponeurotic defects can be repaired via an anterior or a posterior approach, but only the anterior approach will be considered in this book.

ANTERIOR APPROACH APONEUROSIS REPAIR
(Fig 5.5)

Principle

The aponeurosis is approached through a skin incision. It is advanced and sutured to the tarsus or the aponeurotic defect is

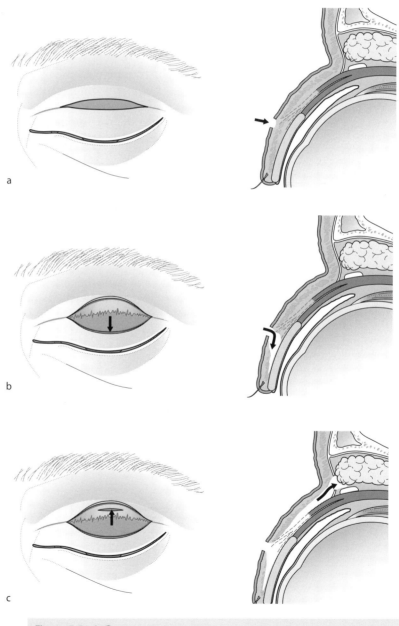

Figure 5.5, A-C

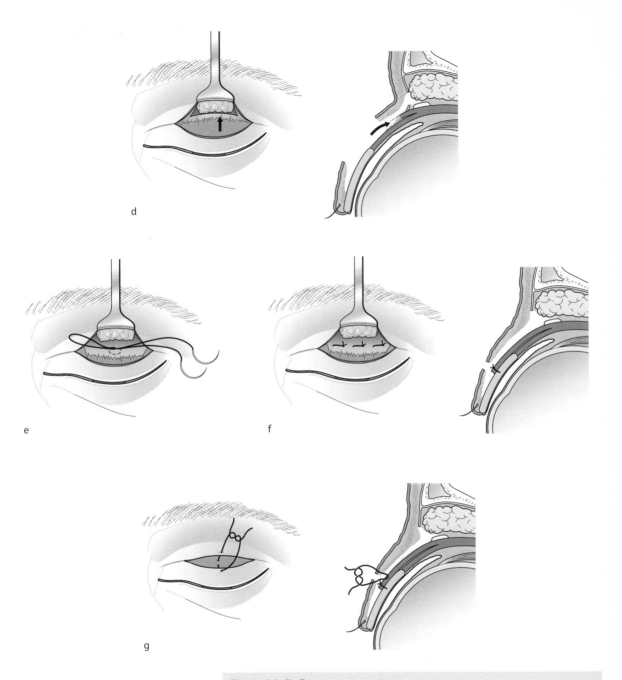

Figure 5.5 D-G

repaired directly. Excess skin can be excised and the skin crease reformed with sutures which pick up the underlying aponeurosis.

Indications

Repair or exploration of an aponeurotic defect, especially if there is excess skin to be excised.

Method

1. Pull the eyebrow skin gently upwards with the finger and mark the skin crease to match the uninvolved side, keeping the skin under light tension. Check this position by reforming the skin crease with open forceps. Preoperatively the position of the skin crease can be assessed by pressing with forceps or a curved piece of wire such as a bent paper clip. Make an incision through the skin with a blade (Fig 5.5a).

2. Pick up the skin on either side of the incision in the centre of the lid with two pairs of toothed forceps and make a cut through the orbicularis muscle with a pair of scissors aimed towards the tarsal plate.

3. Undermine the orbicularis medially and laterally and cut it with scissors along the line of the skin incision.

4. Clean the anterior tarsal surface sufficiently to suture the aponeurosis or levator muscle to it. Stop 2 mm from the lid margin to prevent damage to the lash roots (Fig 5.5b).

5. Dissect the preseptal orbicularis muscle from the lower part of the orbital septum. The septum can be identified by the following:
   a. its attachment to the orbital rim, which can be felt as a firm band when traction is exerted on it.
   b. orbital fat can sometimes be seen behind it.
   c. pressure over the lower lid may help to make the orbital fat more obvious.

6. Open the orbital septum to expose the preaponeurotic fat pad, beneath which is the aponeurosis (Fig 5.5c). This can be seen to move when the patient looks up, if the operation is under local anaesthesia.

7. Examine the levator complex. If there is an aponeurotic disinsertion (Fig 5.5d) advance the healthy aponeurotic tissue and suture it to the tarsus. If there is a defect elsewhere, repair it directly. To correct a disinsertion pass a double-armed long-acting absorbable suture into the anterior tarsal surface at the intended apex of the lid curve and at about the junction of the lower two-thirds with the upper one-third of the tarsus. Pass each needle through healthy aponeurosis and tie the suture with a slip knot (Fig 5.5e).

8. Inspect the lid height and contour. The level should be the same or a little higher than its fellow. Adjust the suture if necessary and then cut it using each arm to suture the aponeurosis to the tarsus on either side of the first central suture (Fig 5.5f).

Note: If the surgery is carried out under general anaesthesia or the levator function is abolished by the local anaesthesia, adjustable sutures can be used (p 107).

9. Excise any excess skin from the upper skin flap.
10. Close the skin and reform the skin crease with 6 '0' absorbable sutures which pass from the edge of the lower skin flap into the aponeurosis and out through the edge of the upper skin flap (Fig 5.5g).

    Note: absorbable sutures are preferable since skin crease sutures may be difficult to remove completely and the scar is buried in the crease.
11. A lower lid traction suture can be used if there is any danger of corneal exposure and the lids left padded for 24–48 hours.

Complications

Lid level too high or too low; contour abnormality; asymmetrical skin crease and upper lid show.

If the lid level, contour and skin crease is seriously wrong the patient can be reoperated straight away. If the lid level is only slightly too high it may respond to eyelid traction. In the immediate post-operative period it is often difficult to judge whether the result will or will not be acceptable, in which case the eyelid should be left alone for healing to occur and any adverse results can be corrected after several months.

LEVATOR RESECTION

The eyelid elevation which can be obtained by shortening the levator complex depends primarily on the levator function. The result required depends on the circumstances, i.e. the diagnosis, Bell's phenomenon, etc. The optimum result in a patient with simple congenital ptosis is for the eyelid levels to be the same in the primary position of gaze, but a lower level may be acceptable in a patient with a partial third nerve palsy, a dry eye or progressive external ophthalmoplegia, etc. A resection of the following amount of aponeurosis and levator muscle should lift the eyelid to an acceptable level:

- Levator function 8–10 mm: 14–18 mm resection
- Levator function 6–7 mm: 18–22 mm resection
- Levator function 4–5 mm: 22–26 mm resection.

These measurements are approximate. They include both aponeurosis and levator muscle and are taken from just below the upper border of the tarsal plate. The extent of the resection is modified by the degree of ptosis; thus 2 mm of ptosis will warrant a lesser resection than 4 mm of ptosis if the levator function is the same. If the superior rectus muscle is weak, the resection should be increased by about 4 mm. The adequacy of the resection can be confirmed at operation. Under general anaesthesia the eyelid should stay at approximately the level that is achieved at operation if the levator function is about 7 mm. If the levator function is better than this the lid will tend to rise postoperatively and to fall if the levator function is worse. Under local anaesthesia the lid should be set 1–2 mm higher to compensate for the paralysis of the orbicularis muscle.

If the patient is mature enough to allow sutures to be manipulated postoperatively, adjustable sutures can be considered. This is particularly useful when general anaesthesia is used in adults and it is difficult to guess what level to set the eyelid e.g. following a post-traumatic upper lid exploration, division of scar and ptosis surgery etc.

ANTERIOR APPROACH LEVATOR RESECTION
(Fig 5.6)

Principle
The levator muscle is approached through a skin incision. The septum is divided and when the preaponeurotic fat is retracted the whole levator complex can be examined directly for any defects. The muscle is shortened and sutured directly to the tarsus. Any excess skin can be excised and the skin crease reformed with interrupted sutures which pick up the underlying levator muscle.

Indications
A ptosis with 4 mm or more of levator function; excess skin needing excision; need for lid exploration e.g. after trauma; maximum levator resection with or without an internal sling; preservation of tarsus and conjunctiva; lash ptosis; entropion; skin crease defect.

Method
Stages 1–6 as for anterior approach aponeurosis repair (see p 96) (Fig 5.6a,b,c).
  7. Dissect the aponeurosis from the tarsus (Fig. 5.6d) and Müller's muscle from the conjunctiva (Fig 5.6ei). Follow this plane to expose the white fascia of the superior suspensory ligament of the fornix and the common sheath between the levator and superior rectus muscles.
     Note: Müller's muscle can be retained if the dissection is carried out at a higher level (Fig 5.6eii). This preserves some sympathetic control of the lid level but is usually only possible with first operations in which Müller's muscle has not been violated. It is less easy to identify the plane under the levator muscle but the rest of the operation is carried out as described below.

8. If the levator complex cannot be advanced sufficiently to lift the lid by the desired amount, cut the medial and lateral attachments (horns) under direct vision. Curve the scissors centrally towards the levator muscle to avoid the trochlea medially and the lacrimal gland laterally (Fig 5.6f).

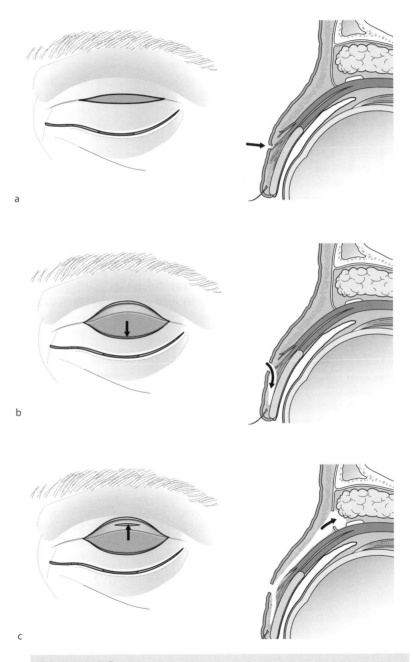

Figure 5.6, A-C

9. Try to preserve Whitnall's ligament and advance the levator muscle under it (Fig. 5.6g).

   Note: If the levator muscle is not separated from Whitnall's ligament, the muscle and the ligament can be sutured directly to the tarsus to act as an internal sling in cases with poor levator function as an alternative to a brow suspension.

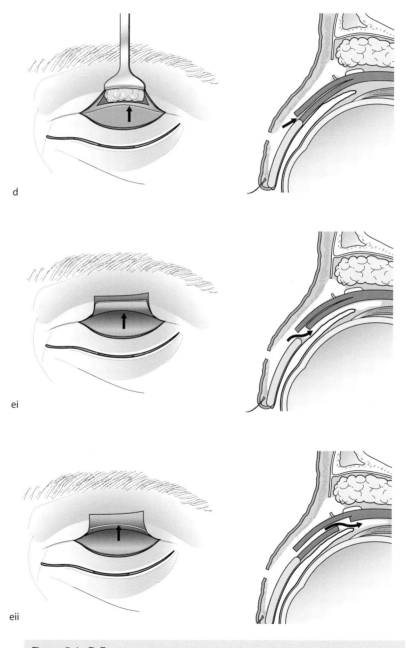

d

ei

eii

Figure 5.6, D-E

This creates a relatively static lid with a marked degree of asymmetry on downgaze in unilateral cases but it is an effective way of raising the lid. The elevation can be further increased if the upper part of the tarsus is resected.

10. Pass a double-armed 6 '0' long-acting absorbable suture into the anterior tarsal surface at the intended apex of the lid curve. Measure the aponeurosis and levator to be resected and pass

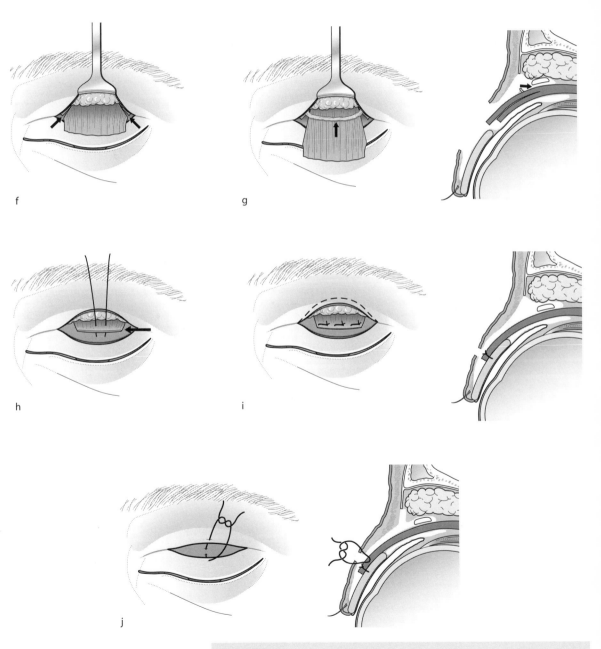

Figure 5.6, F-J

each needle of the suture through the centre of the levator muscle just above the site of the planned resection. Tie the suture with a slip knot and cut the muscle (Fig 5.6h).

11. Check the height and curve of the lid and adjust the suture if necessary. Cut the suture and use each arm to suture the muscle to the tarsus on either side of the central first suture (Fig 5.6i).
12. Thin the lower skin flap by excising a strip of orbicularis muscle.
13. Excise any excess skin from the upper skin flap.
14. Close the skin and reform the crease with 6 '0' absorbable sutures which pass from the edge of the lower skin flap, into the levator muscle, and out through the edge of the upper skin flap (Fig 5.6j). These sutures can be left to absorb in children but are usually removed in adults after about 10 days to prevent suture reactions.
    Note: If the lid has been lifted sufficiently to run a risk of corneal exposure or there is some limitation of ocular motility increasing this risk it may be wise to protect the cornea as follows:

Lower lid traction (Frost) suture (Fig 5.7)

15. Place a 4 '0' nonabsorbable suture in the lower lid margin through the grey-line opposite the point of maximum height of the upper lid. Pull the lower lid up to protect the cornea and tape the suture to the brow (Fig 5.7a).
16. Remove the Frost suture preferably after 24 hours but it can be left for 48 hours. Keep the lids padded until then to allow postoperative swelling to subside. If there is an increased risk of corneal exposure pass the suture through silicone tubing on the skin so that the traction can be reapplied if necessary (Fig 5.7b).

Complications

Corneal exposure; eyelid level too high or too low; conjunctival prolapse; contour abnormality; lash ptosis; entropion; lash eversion and ectropion; poor corneal skin crease.

CORNEAL EXPOSURE

This may occur after any ptosis surgery. The risks are greatest following large levator resections and internal slings, conditions with a poor Bell's phenomenon or weak eyelid closure e.g. third nerve palsies, ocular myopathies; or conditions with a reduced tearfilm e.g. age, dry eye syndromes. Corneal exposure can be treated prophylactically with a lower lid traction suture at the end of operation (Fig 5.7). Use lubricant drops and ointment as frequently as necessary. If the cornea does not respond, the lower lid traction suture can be reinserted. This can be achieved without putting the suture into the skin, which can be particularly helpful for children. Stick a number of pieces of tape to the lid skin after cleaning it with a solvent and/or painting it with Benzylbenzoin. Incorporate a traction suture in the

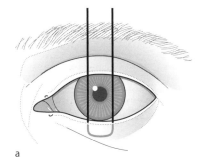

a

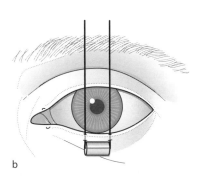

b

Figure 5.7

pieces of tape and reinforce this by adding more pieces of tape. Pull up the traction suture and tape it to the brow. If the cornea will not tolerate the exposure despite these measures the lid must be lowered.

EYELID TOO HIGH

EARLY

The lid can be lowered by releasing or removing adjustable sutures if they have been used. Alternatively the wound can be opened and the levator muscle resutured with 'hang back' sutures if necessary. Traction on the eyelashes and eyelid margin can control the lid level from rising more than it has done already but by itself will not usually correct a significant established lid retraction.

ESTABLISHED

The management is the same as for any lid retraction (p 196).

EYELID TOO LOW

Leave for at least three and preferably six months and then reoperate using the same criteria for assessment as for a new case.

CONJUNCTIVAL PROLAPSE

This usually occurs because the superior suspensory ligament of the fornix, which is the extension of the common sheath between the levator and superior rectus muscles, has been cut when undermining the levator complex. It usually resolves spontaneously provided lubricant ointment is applied to the prolapsed conjunctiva. In adults it may be possible to reposition the prolapse under the lid with a squint hook to help the oedema to settle. If there has been no resolution after several days or weeks the prolapse can be repositioned using Pang-type sutures through the lid (see defective skin crease). Alternatively the excess conjunctiva can be excised and the edges allowed to retract.

CONTOUR ABNORMALITY: OR POSTERIOR APPROACH UPPER LID RETRACTOR RECESSION

Slight peaking can be corrected with a localised tenotomy (p 196). A mild droop can be corrected with a localised Fasanella Servat/tarsectomy type procedure. A severe contour deformity is best managed by exploring the lid and adjusting the resected levator muscle as appropriate.

LASH PTOSIS AND ENTROPION

This is usually caused by failure to pull up the pretarsal flap of skin and orbicularis muscle and to reform the skin crease adequately. It can be corrected with an anterior lamella reposition type of upper lid entropion procedure (p 42).

LASH EVERSION AND ECTROPION

This is usually caused by pulling up the pretarsal flap of skin and orbicularis muscle too much and reforming the skin crease too aggressively. An early mild lash ectropion can often be corrected by removing the skin crease reforming sutures and applying massage or eyelid traction. If this fails the anterior lamella can be undermined to the lash root. The upper lid retractors may need to be recessed a little from the tarsus. The preseptal skin and muscle may need to be advanced a little and the skin crease gently reformed.

DEFECTIVE SKIN CREASE

PROPHYLAXIS

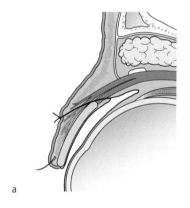

a

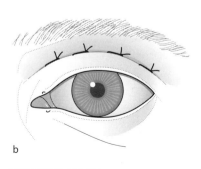

b

Figure 5.8

Apart from the eyelid level and contour, the most important measurement for eyelid symmetry in the primary position of gaze is the 'upper lid show' or amount of eyelid which is visible between the eyelashes and the edge of the overhanging fold of upper lid skin. This depends on the position of the skin crease, the height of the eyelid and the amount of skin in the upper lid. If the eyelids achieve the same height and there is the same amount of skin in both lids the skin crease levels should be symmetrical to give a symmetrical upper lid show. If there is less upper lid skin in the operated eyelid the skin crease needs to be set lower to produce a symmetrical upper lid show. If there is more upper lid skin, the skin crease can be set higher or the excess skin can be excised. If it is intended to only partially correct the ptosis and leave the lid lower than the other side the skin crease should be set a little low. An upper lid show that is greater on one side than the other gives the optical impression of a ptosis on the side with the higher skin crease even if the lid levels are almost equal. A postoperative asymmetry of the upper lid show and skin crease can be corrected as follows:

1. **Pang sutures**. Pass double-armed 4 '0' absorbable sutures through the lid from the conjunctival surface above the tarsal plate and tie them tightly in the prospective skin crease (Fig. 5.8). The sutures create fibrosis which increases the longer they are left but may cause a granuloma, and are therefore best removed after 2–3 weeks if they have not been absorbed. If Pang sutures fail, proceed as below.
2. **Anterior approach skin crease reformation** (see Fig 5.6j)

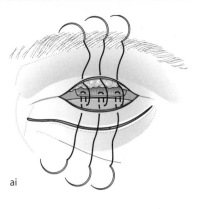

ai

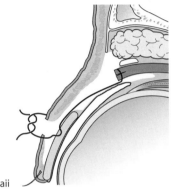

aii

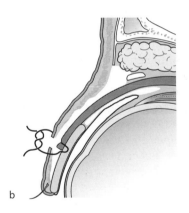

b

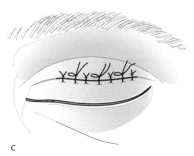

c

Figure 5.9

a. Make a skin crease incision where it is hoped to reform the crease.

b. Identify the lid retractors as in an anterior approach levator resection.

c. Thin the edge of the skin flaps by excising a strip of orbicularis muscle.

d. Close the skin with sutures, which pick up the lid retractors and recreate the crease (see Fig 5.6j).

ADJUSTABLE SUTURES FOR PTOSIS (OR LID RETRACTION) (Fig 5.9)

Principle

The aponeurosis and/or levator muscle are advanced or recessed by tightening or releasing adjustable sutures which pass from the retractor into the tarsal plate and out through the skin edges. The skin crease is reformed separately so that adjusting the sutures does not open the wound. The extent of the surgery obviously depends on the degree of ptosis or lid retraction, the state of the levator muscle etc.

Indications

Any situation where it is likely to be desirable to adjust the lid level or contour in the early postoperative period, e.g. when ptosis or lid retraction surgery has been carried out under general anaesthesia or under local anaesthesia which has paralysed the upper lid movement. Adjustable sutures are particularly valuable when the ptosis or lid retraction surgery is carried out at the same time as other procedures, e.g. correction of trauma, tumour surgery etc. Their use is dependent on the patient being mature enough to allow postoperative suture manipulation.

Method

Stages 1–8 as for anterior approach levator resection.

9. Try to preserve Whitnall's ligament. Free the levator muscle from it if appropriate so that the levator complex can be advanced or recessed (see Fig 5.6g).

10. Pass each needle of a double-armed 5 '0' long-acting absorbable suture through the levator muscle complex or aponeurosis a little higher than you anticipate will be required with the sutures about 3 mm apart. Then pass each needle into the anterior tarsal surface at about the intended skin crease level, keeping the sutures about 3 mm apart. Pass one needle through the edge of the lower skin/muscle flap and the other needle through the edge of the upper skin/muscle flap (Fig 5.9a).

11. Pull on the sutures to advance the levator complex or aponeurosis and raise the lid (Fig 5.9b). Release the sutures and pull on the lid to lower it. The sutures should have been placed high enough

so that when they are pulled the lid level ends up a little higher than you anticipate will be required to correct the ptosis.

12. Place two more similar sutures on either side of the first central suture.
13. Reform the skin crease by suturing the skin edges to the tarsus. Use interrupted 6 '0' absorbable sutures placed between the adjustable sutures. Preferably use sutures of a different colour so they can be easily identified. Ensure that the preaponeurotic fat is free and comes down to the suture line to help maintain the skin crease.
14. Tie the three adjustable sutures with a slip knot (Fig 5.9c).
15. Pad the eye closed using a lower lid traction suture if required.
16. The sutures can be adjusted and tied at any time from 4–24 hours postoperatively. If the suture ends are left relatively long the knots can be unpicked with fine forceps and a further adjustment made up to 5–7 days later or after an even longer period.
17. Remove the sutures at 4 weeks if they have not absorbed or been removed before.

Complications

These are the same as for an anterior approach levator resection but suture reactions are more common.

Adjustable sutures tied in the skin crease can set up a sterile inflammatory reaction as part of the absorption process or they can become infected. In both cases the sutures should be removed.

A lid which is too high can be lowered by early removal of the sutures followed by eyelid traction etc.

The eyelid level and contour can be improved by late adjustment of the sutures as described under method 16.

BROW SUSPENSION/FRONTALIS SLING (Fig 5.10)

Principle

The frontalis muscle normally lifts the eyebrow and contributes to eyelid elevation. This action of lifting the eyelid is enhanced by connecting the frontalis muscle and eyebrow to the eyelid with a subcutaneous 'sling' for which various materials can be used. A unilateral sling will always produce an asymmetrical result on downgaze. This does not matter if the sling is carried out for functional reasons, e.g. to prevent amblyopia, etc. For a definitive cosmetic procedure it is preferable to do a bilateral suspension with weakening or division of the other levator muscle if this is normal (see below). Both eyelids are then dependent on the frontalis muscle but such a bilateral procedure should only be carried out if there is a good chance of a symmetrical result.

Indications

Ptosis with less than 4 mm of levator function; the prevention of amblyopia in an infant with severe ptosis in whom an assessment of levator function is not possible; following a levator excision.

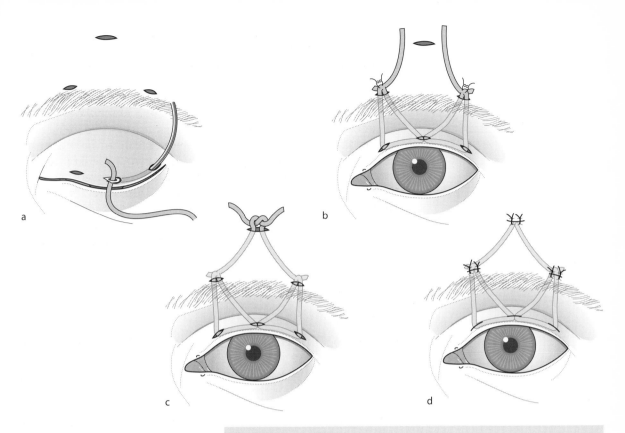

Figure 5.10

- Crawford frontalis sling: autogenous fascia lata.
- Fox pentagon: nonautogenous material.

Suspensory materials:
- Autogenous
  - fascia lata, temporalis fascia
- Nonautogenous
  - integrateable e.g. mersilene mesh, Gortex
  - nonintegrateable e.g. supramid or prolene suture, silicone rod etc.

Autogenous fascia lata is the best material for a sling but needs to be harvested, which limits its use in very young children and in the old and infirm. There is little risk of infection, absorption and breakage such as may occur with foreign materials. It can be used with any technique, but that described by Crawford gives excellent control of lid level and contour. The Crawford technique using fascia lata is therefore the procedure of choice for a brow suspension/frontalis sling procedure if there is no contraindication to harvesting fascia.

Nonautogenous material must be used in very young children who are too small for fascia lata to be harvested. It is also used in old patients and those in whom a general anaesthetic may be contraindicated such as patients with ocular myopathies. A nonintegrateable material such as supramid is very helpful for the prevention of amblyopia. The standard management and prophylaxis of amblyopia with patching of the good eye, refraction and glasses if necessary, should also be instigated. An integrateable material such as a 3 mm strip of Mersilene mesh is valuable for a more permanent ptosis correction if there is a contraindication to the use of fascia lata.

A Fox pentagon is the procedure of choice with foreign material. Less material is required than with the Crawford technique. The insertion is quick and easy and the stab incisions are in different positions to the Crawford technique. Autogenous fascia lata and the Crawford technique can therefore be used at a subsequent operation if a child has had foreign material and a Fox pentagon as an initial procedure to prevent amblyopia and then later requires further surgery. The leg is usually large enough to take fascia lata by about the age of three and a half years.

A. CRAWFORD BROW SUSPENSION/ FRONTALIS SLING (Fig 5.10)

Method

1. Make a medial, central and lateral horizontal skin mark on the eyelid about 2–3 mm from the lash line. The skin crease will form here. If a higher crease is desired, the marks must be raised, but this will reduce the sling's mechanical advantage in raising the lid. Make two marks just above the eyebrow, one vertically above and a little lateral to the lateral eyelid mark, and the other vertically above and a little medial to the medial eye mark. Make a forehead mark above and between these two brow marks to complete an isosceles triangle. Preferably mark and operate on both eyelids at the same time to ensure symmetry.
2. Make stab incisions through all the marks, widening the three forehead incisions a little.
3. Use a Wright's fascial needle to pass each strip of fascia as shown in the diagram (Fig 5.10a).
   Note: a. The fascia should be deep to the orbicularis muscle and superficial to the tarsal plate and orbital septum.
   b. It may be easier to pass the needle between the lid margin incisions if the pretarsal muscle has been partially freed from the underlying tarsus with Westcott scissors.
   c. It is important to ensure that the needle does not catch the periosteum as this will tether the fascia and prevent the frontalis muscle from lifting the lid.
4. Pull up the two triangles of fascia to give a symmetrical lid curve. If there is a normal Bell's phenomenon, raise the lid level as high as possible but stop if it reaches the limbus or if the lid starts to leave the globe. Tie the fascia and reinforce the knot with a 6 '0' absorbable suture (Fig 5.10b).

5. Pull one fascial strip from each eyebrow incision through the forehead incision. Tie the strips together (Fig 5.10c) and reinforce the knot with a 6 '0' absorbable suture.

6. Close the forehead and eyebrow incisions with 6 '0' nylon sutures (buried 6 '0' absorbable sutures can be used in a child). Leave the eyelid incisions open (Fig 5.10d).

7. If required tape a lower lid traction suture to the brow. Remove it at the first dressing 12–48 hours postoperatively. Remove the skin sutures at 5 days.

8. Use lubricant and antibiotic drops and ointment as after any ptosis operation but emphasise the need for ointment at night to prevent corneal exposure problems.

B. FOX PENTAGON (Fig 5.11)

Method

1. Make two skin marks between those that would be made for the Crawford technique. Check the skin crease and lid contour by pushing on these marks with forceps and adjust them as necessary. Make the three higher incisions as for the Crawford technique (Fig 5.11a).

2. Make stab incisions through the marks. Only the central forehead incision needs to be widened.

3. Push an appropriate needle, e.g. Wright's fascial needle or the needles that are supplied with a double-armed prolene or supramid suture, through the incisions and pull the material deep to the orbicularis muscle. If small pieces of a suture are passed under the sling at each incision before it is tightened, the sling can be removed or replaced easily if the contour etc. is incorrect (Fig 5.11b).

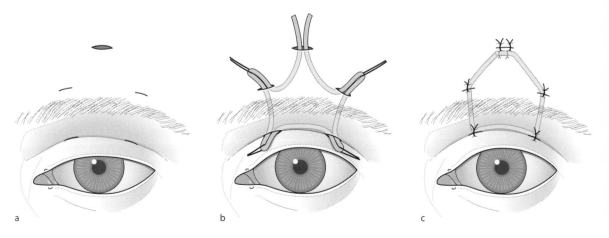

a   b   c

Figure 5.11

4. Pull up the sling as in the Crawford technique. Tie and bury it deeply below the forehead incision.

5. Close the forehead incision carefully (Fig 5.11c) and use a lower lid traction suture etc. as for the Crawford technique.

6. Give systemic antibiotics if foreign material has been used and manage as with the Crawford procedure.

Complications of brow suspension/ frontalis sling procedures

These are the same as for other ptosis operations. If the eyelid is too high or it must be lowered because of corneal exposure problems, any of the sling materials can be released a little or easily removed in the early postoperative period. With autogenous fascia or integrate-able materials once they have become incorporated in the tissues it may be difficult to remove them completely. The sling material can be cut. If it is desirable to keep the skin crease in the same place cut the material relatively high on the lid away from the skin crease. If it is desirable to raise the skin crease, cut the material low near the skin crease at the level at which the new skin crease is required. The lid often needs to be put on traction and a considerable amount of free-ing of adhesions may be required to get the eyelid to drop.

Nonintegrateable material can be easily removed at any time and the lid lowered as the material does not set up the same fibrous tissue reaction as integrateable material.

Granulomas will occur with any integrateable material if it is exposed. The area of the granuloma needs to be excised as widely as possible and the tissue closed. The eyelid level is often unaffected by this because of the fibrous tissue reaction but if the lid does drop the patient can undergo reoperation when everything has settled.

LEVATOR DIVISION OR EXCISION (Fig 5.12)

Principle

The action of the levator muscle is reduced or abolished by dividing or excising it.

Indications

The abolition of aberrant eyelid movements, e.g. jaw-winking; to promote the use of the frontalis muscle and create symmetry in patients undergoing a bilateral brow suspension procedure for a unilateral ptosis.

Method

1. Place a traction suture in the tarsus, evert the lid over a Desmarres' retractor and make a conjunctival incision just above the upper border of the tarsus.

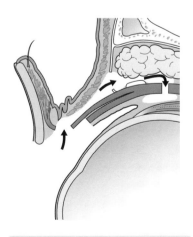

Figure 5.12

2. Cut through Müller's muscle, identify and cut the distal fibres of the aponeurosis, and open the orbital septum to expose the preaponeurotic fat.
3. Identify and clean the belly of the levator muscle above Whitnall's ligament. Pass two squint hooks under the muscle and clamp, cut and cauterise it, letting the proximal end retract into the orbit. This will weaken the muscle, but to abolish aberrant movements it is better to excise a large section of the muscle, i.e. about 10 mm. Even then, fibrous adhesions will reform and allow some aberrant movement to recur after a few weeks.
4. Close the conjunctiva with a continuous 6 '0' absorbable suture.
5. Proceed with a bilateral brow suspension/frontalis sling.

Eyelid reconstruction and tumour management

6

EYELID RECONSTRUCTION

The repair of any eyelid defect depends on its size and position and the state of the surrounding tissues. The approach is similar whatever the cause. With a partial thickness defect of either the anterior or posterior lamella, try a direct closure first and if this is impossible use a flap or graft. Alternatively, consider allowing a defect to granulate and heal by second intention. With a full-thickness defect try a direct closure first and if this is impossible do a lateral cantholysis and free the orbital septum. If closure is still impossible, choose a combination of a flap and graft as appropriate. One lamella should have blood supply to support the other lamella, i.e. a flap and a graft or two flaps can be sutured together but not two grafts.

ANTERIOR LAMELLA DEFECTS

DIRECT SKIN CLOSURE (Fig 6.1)

A partial thickness wound should always be sutured as vertically as possible to reduce the chance of an ectropion or of lagophthalmos (Fig 6.2a,b). Eyelid skin heals so well that this does not usually produce an unacceptable scar. If the localised scar causes symptoms or is unsightly, a Z-plasty can be performed (p 73).

SKIN FLAPS (Figs 6.2, 6.3, 6.4, 6.5)

If the defect cannot be closed directly with undermining, a local skin flap usually gives a better cosmetic result than a graft, e.g. local advancement flap (Fig 6.2a,b), O-Z plasty (Fig 6.3a,b), bilobed flap (Fig 6.4a,b), rhomboid (Fig 6.5a b), transposition flap (see Figs 6.14, 6.15, 6.16, 6.17, 6.18) etc.

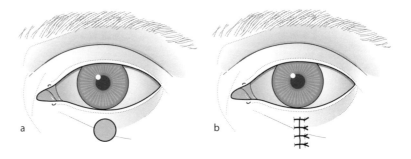

Figure 6.1

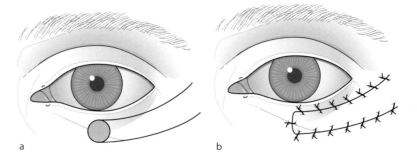

Figure 6.2

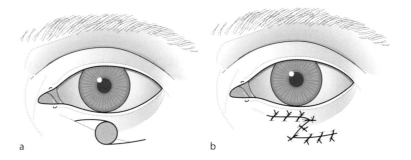

Figure 6.3

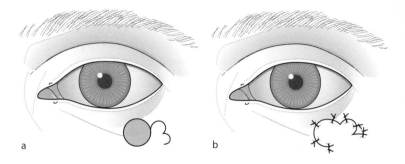

Figure 6.4

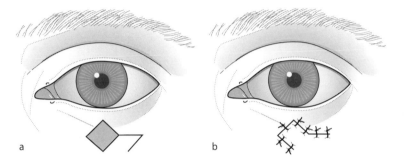

Figure 6.5

SKIN GRAFTS (See Chapter 2)

A full-thickness graft is preferable to a split-thickness graft for defects of both lids unless not enough full-thickness skin is available, e.g. in burns, or the graft bed is unfavourable, e.g. periosteum.

LAISSEZ-FAIRE

Allowing an anterior lamella defect to granulate and heal by secondary intention is sometimes valuable especially if there is not much spare skin available e.g. if the apex of a flap necroses etc.

POSTERIOR LAMELLA DEFECTS

Posterior lamella defects, like anterior lamella defects, can be closed directly or with a flap or graft or they can be allowed to granulate as in the bare sclera technique. Conjunctival Z-plasty flaps are described here. A tarsoconjunctival flap is described on p 126. The following posterior lamella grafts may be used: labial or buccal mucosa (p 16), hard palate mucosa (p 18), sclera or a scleral substitute (p 22 and 23), tarsus (p 15), ear cartilage (p 22) and nasal septal cartilage with its mucoperichondrium (p 20). The technique of a posterior lamella graft and eversion of the lid margin is described in Chapter 3, and the technique of fornix-deepening sutures and a mucous membrane graft is described on p 224.

SYSTEM FOR POSTERIOR LAMELLA DEFECTS (SYMBLEPHARON)

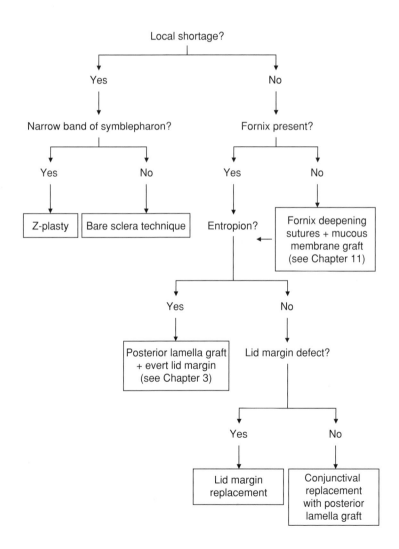

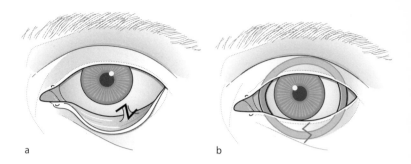

Figure 6.6

CONJUNCTIVAL Z-PLASTY (Fig 6.6)

Principle

Two flaps of conjunctiva are transposed to lengthen a narrow scar at the expense of shortening the conjunctiva at right angles to it (**see Fig 4.15**).

Indications

A narrow band of symblepharon.

Method

1. Make an incision along the line of the scar.
2. Make another incision from each end of this first incision at 60° to it and of approximately the same length (Fig 6.6a).
3. Excise the scar.
4. Transpose the flaps and suture them with a 6 '0' absorbable suture.
5. Insert a ring conformer of a suitable size to maintain the fornix but which still allows the lids to close (Fig 6.6b).

BARE SCLERA TECHNIQUE (Fig 6.7)

Principle

A band of scarred conjunctiva is dissected off the globe. It is retained in the fornix with a ring conformer and the bare sclera is allowed to granulate.

Indications

A symblepharon due to a localised scar which is too diffuse for a Z-plasty but which does not require a mucosal graft.

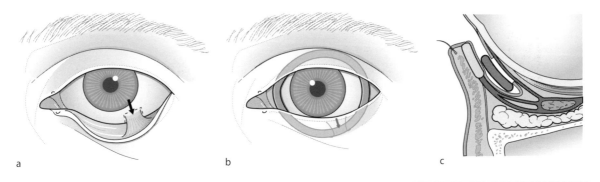

Figure 6.7

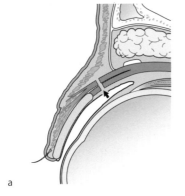

a

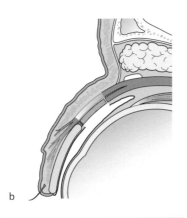

b

Figure 6.8

Method

1. Dissect the scarred conjunctiva from the globe and remove all the scar tissue (Fig 6.7a).
2. Insert a ring conformer or shell to create the fornix and retain this until the sclera has become covered with conjunctiva (Fig 6.7b,c).

   Note: If a scleral ring is not available, the recessed conjunctiva can be sutured to the sclera directly or to the orbital rim with fornix deepening sutures. The bare area will conjunctivalise but the fornix is usually better reformed if a scleral ring or shell is used.

CONJUNCTIVAL REPLACEMENT POSTERIOR LAMELLA GRAFT (Figs 6.8, 6.9)

Principle

The posterior lamella of the lid is lengthened with a graft inserted above the tarsus in the upper lid and below the tarsus in the lower lid. If there is no entropion, there is no need to interfere with the stability of the lid margin by cutting into the tarsus.

Conjunctiva is most effectively replaced with a graft of conjunctiva or tarsus or failing that of mucosa, e.g. labial, buccal, hard palate or nasal septal cartilage with its mucoperichondrium. Ear cartilage, sclera or a scleral substitute can be used but depends on providing a scaffold over which healthy remaining conjunctiva can grow. Until this happens the surface of the graft is bare and relatively rough which makes them less suitable for upper lid posterior lamella replacement.

Indications

Shortage of the posterior lamella of the lid with no associated entropion.

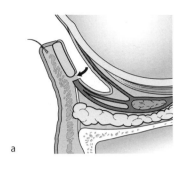

a

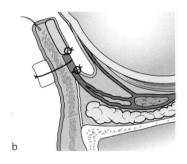

b

Figure 6.9

Method

1. Make an incision at the attached border of the tarsus (Figs 6.8a, 6.9a).
2. Free the conjunctiva, and lid retractors if required, until the posterior lamella shortage is well overcorrected.
3. Suture a graft of mucosa, sclera, or a scleral substitute, tarsus or cartilage between the recessed conjunctiva and lid retractors and the previously attached border of the tarsus with an absorbable suture or a continuous 6 '0' nylon pull-out suture (Fig 6.8b).
4. Suture the graft to its bed with 1–2 double-armed 4 '0' long-acting absorbable sutures tied over bolsters on the skin (Fig 6.9b).
5. Put the lid on traction with a suture through the lid margin.
6. Remove the traction suture after 48 hours and the bolsters after 5 days.

    Note: this technique is similar to lengthening the lid retractors (p 196) but the graft is used primarily to lengthen the conjunctiva and posterior lamella, and the lid retractors are only divided if necessary.

Complications

Corneal abrasion. Remove any sutures or knots abrading cornea. Give antibiotic ointment and consider a bandage contact lens.

LID MARGIN REPLACEMENT POSTERIOR LAMELLA GRAFT

Principle

A posterior lamella graft which reforms the lid margin needs to be stiff for support and mucosal lined for comfort. It is always preferable to repair a defect with similar tissue i.e. like for like. Tarsus is therefore good and can be taken as a free tarsal graft usually from the contralateral upper lid (p 15) or as a tarsomarginal graft which gives a stable lid margin (p 15). Other alternatives include nasal septal cartilage with its attached mucoperichondrium (p 20) and hard palate mucosa (p 18).

Indications

Shortage of posterior lamella involving the lid margin.

Method

These are described as part of the eyelid reconstruction procedures in which they are used e.g. tarsal and tarsomarginal grafts in 'Skin mobilization and posterior lamella reconstruction' (p 123); nasal septal cartilage and hard palate mucosa in 'Lower lid bridge flap' (p 130) etc.

FULL-THICKNESS EYELID DEFECTS

SYSTEM FOR REPAIR OF FULL-THICKNESS EYELID DEFECTS

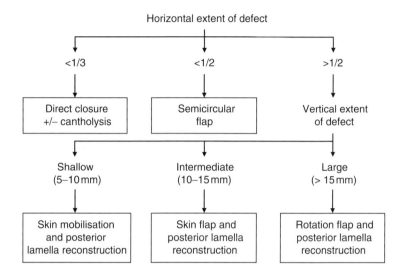

DIRECT CLOSURE (See Fig 2.6)

Method – see Chapter 2

LATERAL CANTHOLYSIS (Fig 6.10)

Method

1. Make a small horizontal incision between the two limbs of the lateral canthal tendon.
2. Through this incision separate the skin and conjunctiva from the appropriate limb using sharp pointed scissors.
3. Put tension on the eyelid that is being repaired and cut the appropriate limb, leaving the other limb of the tendon intact (Fig 6.10a,b).
4. Free the orbital septum as required to obtain satisfactory closure of the defect.
5. Close the conjunctiva to the skin if the cantholysis wound is large.

'SEMICIRCULAR' FLAP (TENZEL) (Fig 6.11)

Method

1. Carry out a lateral cantholysis of the appropriate limb of the lateral canthal tendon (Fig 6.10).

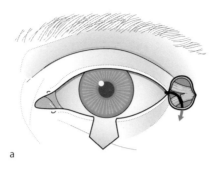
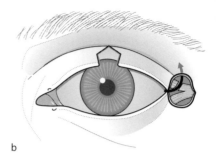

a   b

Figure 6.10

2. Cut a 'semicircular' flap of skin and orbicularis muscle which is high-arched, i.e. the vertical diameter (approximately 22 mm) is more than the horizontal diameter (approximately 18 mm). The incision should keep within the periorbital skin and should not extend laterally beyond the lateral part of the eyebrow (Fig 6.11a,b).

   Note: the lids are not denervated since the branches of the seventh nerve run mainly lateral to this incision and the terminal fibres turn almost vertically to supply the orbicularis muscle.

3. Free the orbital septum, mobilise the conjunctiva, and pull the lid medially to approximate the wound edges. This is much easier with this improved exposure than via a small lateral cantholysis incision.

4. Carry out a direct closure.

5. Create a new lateral canthus with a 4 '0' nonabsorbable vertical mattress suture which suspends the reformed segment of lid from the intact limb of the lateral canthal tendon (Fig 6.11c).

   Note: it is very important in a lower lid reconstruction that the reformed lid is under enough tension to prevent an ectropion.

6. Close the orbicularis muscle with absorbable sutures and the skin with silk, which should be removed at 5 days. The conjunctiva and skin at the reconstructed lid margin should be sutured with a continuous nylon or absorbable suture. The vertical mattress suture should be tied over bolsters and removed at 10 days (Fig 6.11d).

SKIN MOBILISATION AND POSTERIOR LAMELLA RECONSTRUCTION (Fig 6.12)

Principle

Excess skin in an eyelid can often be mobilised to cover a posterior lamella graft without resorting to a formal skin flap. The best posterior

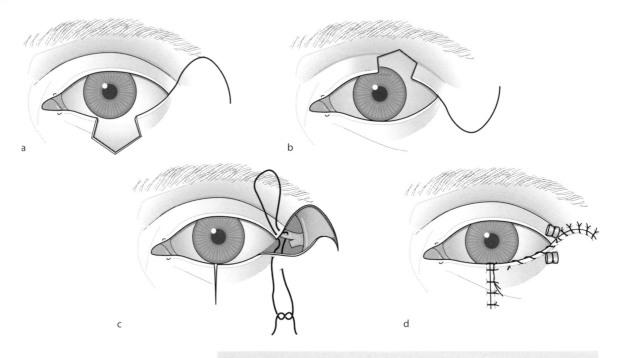

a   b

c   d

Figure 6.11

lamella replacement is tarsus. This can be taken as a free graft from the upper border of the contralateral upper eyelid, as a tarsomarginal graft, or mobilised on a conjunctival pedicle. For a lower lid marginal defect the tarsoconjunctival pedicle is often brought down from the upper eyelid (see below – Hughes flap).

Indications
A shallow marginal upper eyelid defect (Fig. 6.12a).

Method
1. Measure the lid defect with minimal traction on the wound edges (Fig 6.12b).
2. Evert the contralateral upper lid and excise a piece of tarsal plate with the same measurements from its attached upper border (Fig 6.12c,d). Leave a frill of conjunctiva attached to the tarsal graft for reconstruction of the new eyelid margin. The distal 4 mm of a donor plate must be left to preserve the lid margin.
3. Suture the graft into the defect with partial thickness 6 '0' long-acting absorbable sutures tied on the anterior surface away from the cornea.
4. Mobilise the lid skin as a direct advancement or local flap to cover the anterior surface of the graft (Fig 6.12e,f).
5. Suture the frill of conjunctiva to the skin flap to reconstruct the new lid margin (Fig 6.12g).

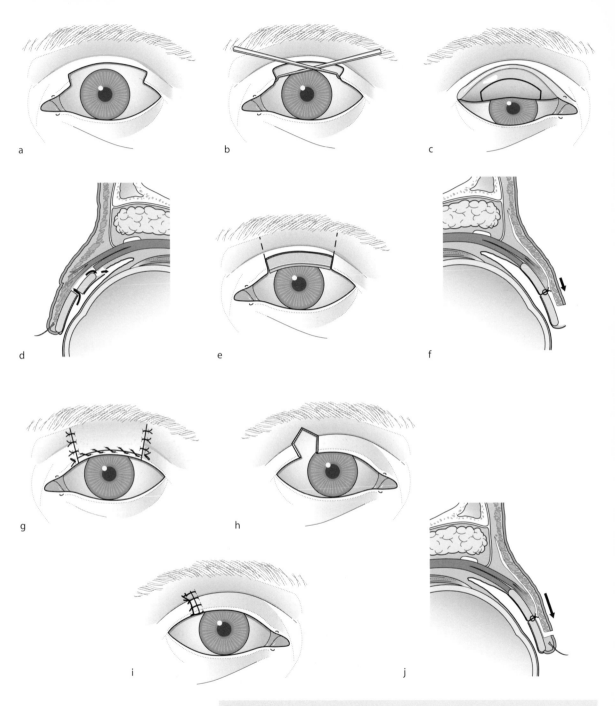

Figure 6.12

Note: a. A tarsomarginal graft from one of the other lids can be used. A full-thickness pentagon of eyelid tissue is resected and the wound closed direct (Fig 6.12h,i). Skin and orbicularis muscle are excised from the graft, leaving tarsus and the lid margin. This gives a stable lid margin (Fig 6.12j) and a relatively large posterior lamella graft vertically if it is taken from an upper eyelid, but its horizontal extent is limited.

b. A nasal septal cartilage graft with its attached mucosa can be used instead of the tarsal graft.

c. It may be possible to fill the defect with tarsus from the same upper lid with or without a conjunctival pedicle. This principle can be extended (see below).

Complications

There is a tendency for the reconstructed area to retract. It should be left a little proud to compensate for this.

TARSOCONJUNCTIVAL FLAP AND SKIN MOBILISATION OR GRAFT (HUGHES) (Fig 6.13)

Principle

A tarsoconjunctival flap is preferable to a free graft for lower lid marginal defects as it provides a vertical lift during the healing phase and can support a skin graft. This is often required since there is less excess skin in a lower lid than in an upper lid. Part of the tarsus from the upper lid is brought down on a conjunctival pedicle and sutured into the lower lid defect. It is covered with mobilised skin or a full-thickness skin graft. At a second operation the conjunctival pedicle is cut and the lower lid margin reconstituted. The integrity of the upper lid margin is retained by leaving the lower 4 mm of the upper tarsal plate intact.

Indications

A marginal defect of the lower lid (Fig 6.13a).

Method

1. Measure the reduced horizontal extent of the lower lid defect after pulling the edges towards each other to compensate for the retraction of the orbicularis muscle and the laxity of the medial and lateral canthal tendons.
2. Evert the upper lid and make a horizontal incision through the tarsus 4 mm above the lid margin and of the same length as the reduced lower lid defect (Fig 6.13b).
3. Make a vertical incision through the tarsus and up into the conjunctiva from each end of the horizontal incision.

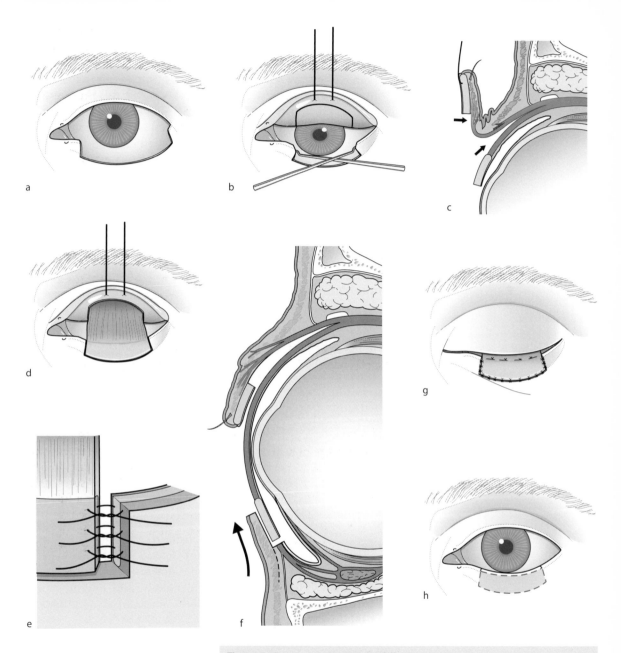

Figure 6.13

4. Dissect and free the tarsoconjunctival flap so that it can be advanced into the lower lid defect under no tension (Fig 6.13c).
5. Suture the flap into the defect with 6 '0' long-acting absorbable sutures (Fig 6.13d,e).

   Note: If the tarsus on the tarsoconjunctival flap is not quite extensive enough to fill the horizontal defect in the lower lid, carry out a lateral cantholysis of the inferior limb of the lateral canthal tendon. If there is no lateral fragment of eyelid which can be mobilised, consider transposing a suitably sized periosteal flap from the lateral orbital rim.

6. Cover the raw anterior surface of the tarsus with locally mobilised skin (Fig 6.13f) or with a suitable full-thickness skin graft as previously described (Fig 6.13g).

7. Divide the conjunctival pedicle when the repair looks well healed – usually after about 3 weeks. Cauterise the new raw lid margin leaving it in line with the remaining resected lid margin remnants. It will granulate to produce a paler smoother lid margin than if it is sutured (Fig 6.13h).

8. The defect in the upper lid is left open to granulate but the upper lid retractors must be freed, recessed and preferably the lid put on traction for 24 hours with subsequent massage if necessary to correct any lid retraction.

Complications

Thickened red lid margin: The risk of this is reduced if the divided flap is cauterised and allowed to granulate. If it occurs, the excess tissue should be excised and the lid margin thinned and cauterised.

Upper lid retraction: If this is not controlled by lash traction and massage, the conjunctival upper lid wound needs to be opened and the retractors formally recessed.

SKIN FLAP AND POSTERIOR LAMELLA GRAFT
(Figs 6.14–6.18)

Principle

A pedicle skin flap is transposed to cover a posterior lamella graft. The site of the flap depends on the position of the defect, e.g. naso-jugal (Fig 6.14) for medial lower lid defects, cheek (Fig 6.15) or upper lid (Fig 6.16) for lateral lower lid defects, forehead above eye-brow (Fig 6.17) for lateral upper lid defects, and midline frontal (Fig 6.18) for medial upper lid defects. This can also be used for lower lid defects.

Indications

An intermediate defect of either eyelid which preferably involves a canthus.

Method

1. The size of the defect is reduced by traction and the posterior lamella is reconstructed, usually with a graft.

2. A suitable site for the flap is selected (Figs 6.14–6.18). The length of the required pedicle is assessed by holding one end of a gauze

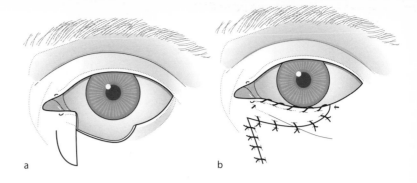

Figure 6.14

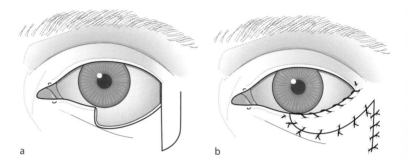

Figure 6.15

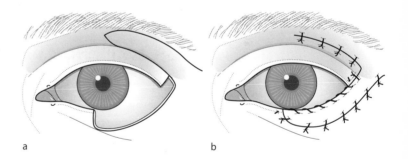

Figure 6.16

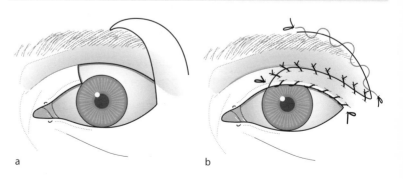

Figure 6.17

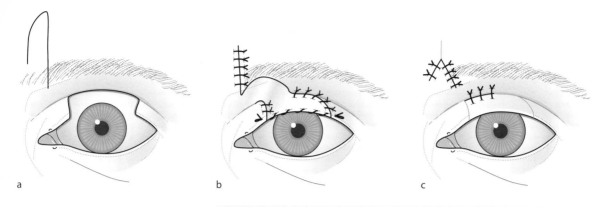

Figure 6.18

swab or piece of suture at the base of the proposed flap and transposing the other end into the defect.

3. The flap is raised and the donor site closed.

4. The flap is thinned as required and sutured over the posterior lamella reconstruction.

5. The base of the pedicle can be restored to its original position after some weeks. This is usually only required if the base of the flap is thick and immobile, as with a forehead flap, or if the flap bridges intact tissue. This classically occurs if the defect is central. A bipedicle upper lid skin flap can be transposed to cover a posterior lamella graft in a central lower lid defect. Conversely, a lower lid pedicle flap can be advanced under the intact lower lid margin to fill an upper lid defect as discussed below (Cutler-Beard).

Complications

Forehead skin tends to be thick and not pliable enough to allow satisfactory mobility of the reconstructed upper lid.

Brow retraction often occurs if a lateral forehead donor site above the eyebrow is closed directly. This can limit closure of the reconstructed eyelids. It can be relieved by skin grafting the donor site but this is not usually cosmetically satisfactorily.

LOWER LID BRIDGE FLAP (CUTLER-BEARD)
(Fig 6.19)

Principle

A flap of lower lid tissue is advanced into a central upper lid defect and can be made to cover a posterior lamella graft. A full-thickness flap of lower lid tissue is mobilised 5 mm below the lid margin. It is passed under the intact bridge of lower eyelid and sutured into the upper lid defect. If the upper lid defect was relatively shallow and the lower lid tissues are lax, they may stretch enough to avoid the need for a posterior lamellar graft. After the flap has been allowed to stretch, it is divided and the lower lid reconstituted.

Indications

A central intermediate defect of the upper eyelid (Fig 6.19a).

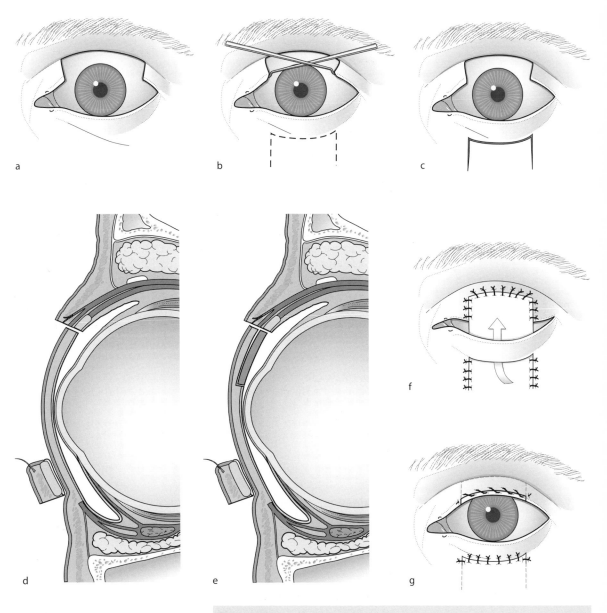

Figure 6.19

Method

1. Measure the reduced horizontal extent of the upper lid defect after pulling the edges towards each other to compensate for the retraction of the orbicularis muscle and laxity of the medial and lateral canthal tendons.

2. Mark this measurement on the lower lid skin 5 mm below the lid margin, and from each end of the mark draw a vertical line downwards (Fig 6.19b).

3. Cut along the skin marks with a blade (Fig 6.19c).

4. Protect the eye with a lid guard and perforate the full thickness of the lid at both ends of the horizontal incision.

5. Transect the lid in the line of the skin incision with scissors, taking care to keep them horizontal.

6. Cut vertically downwards from each end of this incision through the full thickness of the lid, following the skin incisions. Use scissors initially and continue the incision with a blade when over the orbital rim.

7. Pull the flap under the bridge of lower eyelid and suture it in layers into the defect (Fig 6.19d). If the lower fornix conjunctiva cannot be mobilised sufficiently, suture a posterior lamella graft into the upper eyelid defect first and cover it with the flap attaching conjunctiva to the lower border of the graft (Fig 6.19e). It is preferable to use a posterior lamella graft such as tarsus, nasal septal cartilage or hard palate mucosa which has some stiffness and which will support the reconstructed lid margin. If conjunctiva can be mobilised to fill the upper lid defect an ear cartilage, scleral or other similar graft can be sutured between the conjunctiva and orbicularis muscle of the advancement flap as a 'sandwich graft' to provide support (p 22).

8. Suture the skin edges of the advancement flap but do not suture the cut edges of the bridge of lower eyelid (Fig 6.19f).

9. Remove the sutures at 5–7 days.

10. Leave the flap to stretch for 6 weeks to 3 months or longer depending on the circumstances, e.g. laxity of the tissues, extent of the defect, previous radiotherapy, etc.

11. Divide the flap in layers, leaving more conjunctiva than skin attached to the upper lid. It is useful to place a grooved director under the flap and to cut down on it with a blade.

12. Suture the excess conjunctiva round the new lid margin to the skin anteriorly to prevent an entropion. A continuous 6 '0' nylon suture can be used and removed at 5 days.

13. Freshen the inferior border of the lower eyelid bridge and resuture the lower eyelid in layers (Fig 6.19g).

Complications

Necrosis of lower lid bridge. This should not happen if the flap has been cut 5 mm below the lid margin as the marginal artery should be preserved. If it does occur the medial and lateral remnants of the lid margin should be left to granulate until the lower lid advancement flap is ready for division. When the flap is divided, the ends of the lower lid bridge can usually be pulled together with a lateral cantholysis and the lower lid reformed with the advancement flap.

Upper lid entropion. The reconstructed upper lid margin is unstable unless a stiff posterior lamella graft or 'sandwich graft' has been used. An upper lid entropion can be corrected by adding these subsequently. Milder cases can be corrected with an anterior lamella repositioning type of entropion correction.

ROTATION FLAP AND POSTERIOR LAMELLA GRAFT (Figs 6.20, 6.21)

Principle

A large lower lid defect can be corrected with a cheek rotation flap which covers a posterior lamella graft. A large upper lid defect can be corrected by rotating the lower lid into the upper lid defect and reconstructing the lower lid with a cheek rotation flap and posterior lamella graft at a second stage.

Indications

Large vertical upper or lower lid defects.

Method

1. For an upper lid defect mark the lower lid flap to correspond with the upper lid defect (Fig 6.20a).
2. Incise the full thickness of the lower lid but leave a 5 mm pedicle laterally. If necessary, a little more skin can be cut to allow the flap to rotate, but try to preserve the subcutaneous vascular pedicle.
3. Rotate the flap into the upper lid defect and suture it in layers (Fig 6.20b).
4. Leave the flap until it looks healthy, which often takes 3–6 weeks. Cut the pedicle and open the medial upper lid wound enough to suture the rotated lower lid into position (Fig 6.20c).
5. Open the lower lid wound to expose the lower lid defect. The repair is now the same whether the lower lid was used to reconstruct the upper lid or whether the defect only involved the lower lid.
6. Draw a curved line on the skin from the lateral canthus upwards, just missing the lateral eyebrow hairs. Continue upwards over the temple and then curve downwards in front of the ear (Fig 6.21a).
7. Cut the lower limb of the lateral canthal tendon and free the inferior orbital septum to mobilise fully any remnant of lower eyelid lateral to the defect.

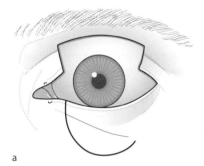

a

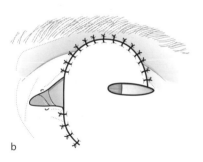

b

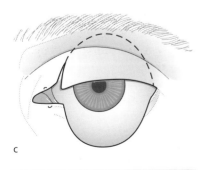

c

Figure 6.20

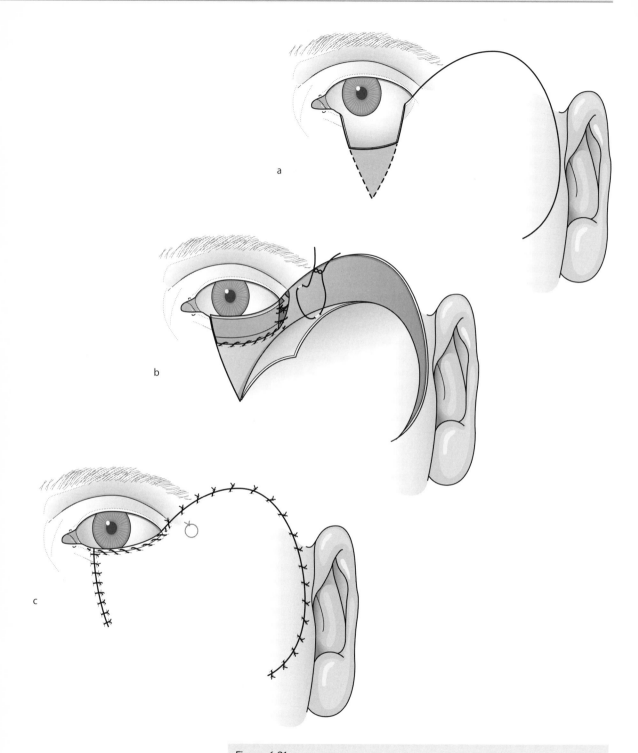

Figure 6.21

8. Start an incision along the skin mark. It should extend through the orbicularis only as far as the lateral orbital rim. After this, the incision should not go any deeper than the subcutaneous fat in order to avoid damage to the facial nerve. Undermine and fully mobilise the flap in this plane and extend the incision as required to fill the defect.

9. Excise a triangle of excess skin below the defect, keeping the medial side of the excision as vertical as possible.

10. Take a graft of nasal septal cartilage and mucosa, or full-thickness oral mucous membrane, and suture it to the remnants of the conjunctiva and tarsus to form a posterior lamella for the new lid.

    Note: a nasal septal cartilage and mucosal graft gives a better lid margin and more support to the lid, but oral mucous membrane is easier to take.

11. Suture the deep surface of the flap to the lateral orbital rim above the new lateral canthus with a nonabsorbable suture. This supports the whole flap and prevents it from sagging (Fig 6.21b).

12. Suture the deep surface of the flap elsewhere to the subcutaneous tissues and to the rest of the orbital rim with absorbable sutures.

13. Close the skin edges with multiple interrupted nonabsorbable sutures. These are removed at 5 days except when they are under tension or at the apex of the suture line medially, where they are left for 10 days.

14. Bring the free mucosa of the graft over the edge of the flap and suture it to the anterior surface of the flap to prevent subsequent shrinkage causing an entropion. A continuous 5 '0' nylon suture can be used and the ends taped or sutured to the skin. This suture is removed at 5 days (Fig 6.21c).

15. The graft may be sutured to the deep surface of the flap with two nonabsorbable sutures which are tied without tension over bolsters on the skin. These are removed after 5–7 days unless they appear to be prejudicing the survival of the flap, when they can be removed earlier.

16. Apply a pressure dressing for 48 hours.

Complications

7th nerve palsy. If the plane of dissection of the cheek rotation flap extends into the orbicularis muscle and is not kept in the subcutaneous fat lateral to the orbital rim (Stage 8) the temporal branch of the facial nerve may be damaged which will limit upper lid closure.

Lower lid retraction. The rotated cheek flap is heavy and as the subcutaneous tissue contracts it tends to retract. This can be minimised by supporting the flap with subcutaneous sutures to the orbital rim (Stage 11). Despite this retraction may occur anyway with time. It may require incision in the flap below the reconstructed lid margin, elevation of the lateral canthus and a full thickness skin graft.

ADDITIONAL REPAIRS

GLABELLAR FLAP (Fig 6.22)

Principle

A V → Y flap is advanced and rotated from the glabellar region.

Indications

Repair of defects involving the medial canthus and the medial part of the upper lid. It is not good for defects extending much below the medial canthus. It can be combined with other procedures, e.g. a lower lid bridge flap.

Method

1. Make an inverted V incision in the midline of the brow with one limb extending down to the defect (Fig 6.22a).
2. Undermine the flap as required, leaving it attached by a broad pedicle across the bridge of the nose.
3. Close the brow defect to make the stem of an inverted Y, using 4 '0' absorbable sutures to support the subcutaneous tissues. This advances the flap and it is rotated on the pedicle across the bridge of the nose (Fig 6.22b).
4. Suture the flap into the defect and to the deep tissues after thinning it as necessary (Fig 6.22c).

Complications

Thick flap. A flap that is too thick may need to be thinned.

Hairy skin. Care needs to be taken to avoid transposing hairy skin into the defect. If it occurs, cryotherapy can be tried.

Medial canthal scars. These may require prolonged pressure and massage to produce a satisfactory result.

LAISSEZ-FAIRE (Fig 6.23)

Principle

A defect is allowed to heal by granulation.

Indications

Medial canthal defects in which it is difficult to obtain satisfactory skin cover, e.g. large medial canthal tumour resections involving both lids, after radiotherapy, etc.

Method

1. Reduce the defect as much as possible by direct skin closure without cutting any flaps.

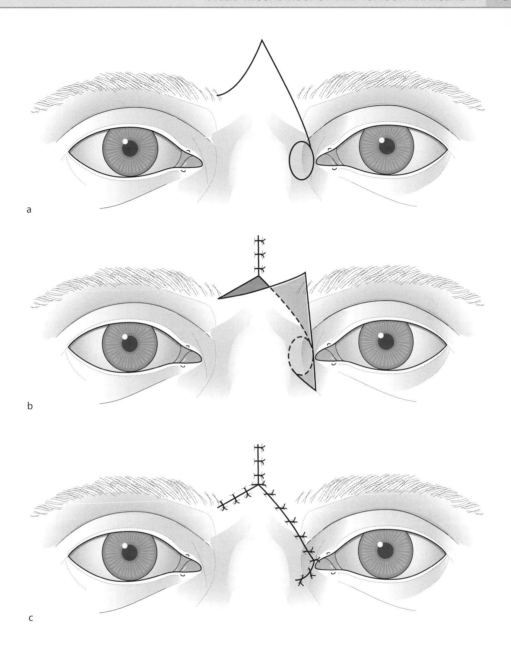

Figure 6.22

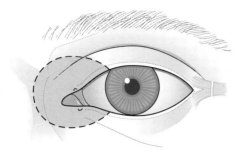

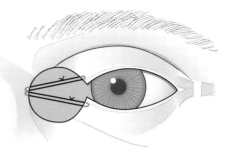

a   b

Figure 6.23

2. Cut the common limb of the lateral canthal tendon from the conjunctival surface to obtain the maximum mobilisation of the lids (Fig 6.23a).
3. Pull the remnants of both upper and lower eyelids medially across the globe and suture them with 4 '0' long-acting absorbable sutures to whatever tissues can be found posteriorly on the medial orbital wall (Fig 6.23b).
4. Pack the wound with Vaseline gauze.
5. Postoperatively, keep the wound clean with daily applications of a swab soaked in an antiseptic solution e.g. Chlorhexidine or half strength Eusol and Paraffin. Allow it to granulate – which can take a very long time..

Complications

Scar contraction. This can lead to eyelid malposition which may subsequently require correction with a skin graft.

EYELID TUMOUR MANAGEMENT

Diagnosis

This is based on history, clinical features, examination, special investigations and pathology. If in doubt about the diagnosis a biopsy should be performed.

Biopsy

Excisional biopsy involves excising the whole lesion and submitting it for histopathology. This is preferable if the lesion is small.

Incisional biopsy involves taking a piece of the lesion preferably with an adjacent edge of presumed normal tissue for comparison.

A full thickness incisional biopsy is indicated when certain rare tumours such as meibomian gland or adenocarcinomas are suspected because of the difficulty of making the histological diagnosis of such tumours with a partial thickness biopsy.

Multiple biopsies can be carried out to assess the extent of the tumour and of associated cytological changes. This may be particularly important when assessing intraepithelial melanocytic changes associated with malignant melanoma or pagetoid spread with meibomian gland or adenocarcinoma. Such multiple biopsies are referred to as conjunctival or skin 'mapping'.

TREATMENT

- Cryotherapy
- Radiotherapy
- Surgical excision and reconstruction
- Antimitotic agents
- Photodyamic therapy.

Cryotherapy, radiotherapy and surgery all have similar cure rates for the common malignant eyelid basal cell carcinomas and squamous cell carcinomas. Meibomian gland, adenocarcinomas and malignant melanomas do better with surgery.

The main disadvantage of cryotherapy and radiotherapy is the lack of histological proof of clearance. This limits their value with morphoeic and other lesions where the tumour margin is uncertain, with lesions involving the fornices and with medial canthal lesions which may extend deeply without giving rise to suspicion.

CRYOTHERAPY

Principle

There is a graded sensitivity of tissues to cold. Pigment cells are destroyed at $-10°C$, hair follicles at $-20°C$ and epithelial cells at $-30°C$. This effect is enhanced if the freeze is rapid, the thaw slow and if the freeze–thaw cycle is repeated.

Indications

Epithelial tumours, e.g. basal and squamous cell carcinomas; benign lesions, e.g. keratoses, papillomas, trichiasis (p 53); small tumours around the canaliculi and lacrimal puncta since the lacrimal drainage apparatus is relatively resistant to cryodamage; when surgery is contraindicated, e.g. when refused, anticoagulants, general health, age, etc; eyelid margin tumours where surgery would be relatively extensive and where radiotherapy could cause keratinisation and discomfort; the basal cell naevoid syndrome and conditions in which multiple basal cell carcinomas develop as there is a limit to how much tissue can be excised and there is always the theoretical risk of inducing malignant change with radiotherapy.

Method

1. Insert a thermocouple under the estimated deepest part of the lesion and preferably a second thermocouple 5–10 mm peripheral to the lesion.
2. Protect the globe and normal skin (p 53).
3. Spray the lesion with liquid nitrogen, including a generous 5–10 mm margin, until both thermocouples record −30°C, and repeat with a double or triple freeze–thaw cycle.

Complications

Depigmentation. Loss of lashes. Thinning of eyelid tissue (see p 53).

RADIOTHERAPY

Principle

Tumour control by destruction of actively dividing cells.

Indications

Sensitive tumours e.g. BCCs and SCCs, as an alternative to surgery or cryotherapy; where surgery is contraindicated, e.g. when refused, anticoagulants, poor general health etc; the lymphomas, myelo-proliferative disorders, Kaposi sarcomas, secondary tumours and for palliation.

Complications

As with cryotherapy, radiotherapy causes depigmentation, loss of lashes, thinning of eyelid tissues. In addition it can cause dryness of the eye from a poor tearfilm and irritation from keratinisation of the conjunctiva or a watering eye from blockage of the lacrimal canali-culi. Other complications, e.g. cataract, should be preventable with modern techniques for shielding the eye.

Recurrences after radiotherapy are difficult to treat surgically as the treated tissue is avascular. There is an increased risk of wound break-down and flap necrosis.

SURGICAL EXCISION

Principle

Removal of the whole lesion which is examined histologically to confirm diagnosis and clearance.

Indications

Any malignant and many benign eyelid tumours which can be removed completely and the defect reconstructed provided the patient understands what is likely to be involved and is prepared and fit enough to undergo surgery. Some tumours such as meibomian gland carcinomas, notoriously mimic other lesions (the masquerade syndrome) and the diagnosis may be impossible unless the whole lesion is available for histology.

Method (Fig 6.24)

A malignant eyelid tumour such as a basal cell carcinoma must be excised with a margin of surrounding healthy tissue, which is usually estimated as 4 mm. The clearance is confirmed histologically as described below, but this 4 mm margin must be added to the tumour dimension when estimating the size of the defect to be repaired. A partial-thickness excision should be carried out with the excision of orbicularis muscle under the tumour if it does not extend to within 4 mm of the eyelid margin and is not fixed to the tarsal plate. A benign lesion does not require such an extensive margin. If a benign lesion is too large to allow a complete excision and simple closure, it can be partially excised in the first instance. The skin is allowed to stretch and the 'serial excision' repeated until the lesion has been removed completely.

A full-thickness excision is required if any malignant tumour extends to within 4 mm of the eyelid margin. It should be shaped as a pentagon, i.e. the excision through the lid margin and tarsal plate should be made at right angles to a tangent to the lid margin (Fig 6.24). When the wound is sutured, the normal curve of the lid is retained and the tension is evenly distributed across the tarsus. With a wedge-shaped resection the tension is maximum at the lid margin, which increases the risk of a notch. It is wise not to excise any apparent excess normal tissue created by the reconstruction, e.g. a 'dog-ear', since this often settles spontaneously and any residual normal tissue may be valuable if further tumour surgery is required.

It may sometimes be reasonable to consider a partial thickness resection of the anterior lamella of the lid with small lesions which are thought to be relatively benign and are closer than 4 mm to the lid margin provided proper facilities exist for histology and adequate follow-up.

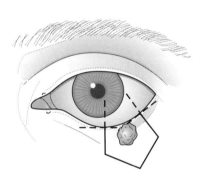

Figure 6.24

CLEARANCE

- Routine histology
- Urgent paraffin section
- Frozen section
- Mohs technique
- Distant spread.

ROUTINE HISTOLOGY (Fig 6.25)

The excised specimen is processed and a series of sections are cut usually horizontally across the long axis of the specimen like cutting a loaf of bread (Fig 6.25). The sections are reported after a variable period of time. The accuracy of the assessment of clearance is directly related to the number of sections examined from different parts of the specimen.

If after a defect has been repaired the routine histology suggests the lesion has not been completely removed, the options are to wait and watch the area, carry out a further excision, or to consider some other treatment such as radiotherapy. Each case should be considered individually but further surgery should be carried out quickly if the tumour is highly malignant and can metastasise or was situated in an area like the medial canthus where it can reach the periosteum and migrate posteriorly without being detected. If it was a relatively benign tumour such as a nodular basal cell carcinoma, and occurred in the centre of the eyelid where it can easily be kept under observation, the area can be observed since many apparently incompletely excised basal cell carcinomas do not recur.

URGENT PARAFFIN SECTION

The technique of routine histology can be speeded up dramatically and the sections read after 24–48 hours. The eyelid remnants can be temporarily sutured or padded closed over the eye to protect it until the results are known. The reconstruction can then proceed as a second stage once clearance has been confirmed. This can be of great value in eyelid tumour management as paraffin sections allow more accurate assessment than frozen sections. This is particularly important with meibomian gland carcinomas and malignant melanomas.

FROZEN SECTION (Fig 6.26)

Frozen sections can be carried out at the time of surgery. They are quick and particularly valuable when the number of sections that need to be examined is kept to a minimum e.g. when assessing the medial and/or lateral clearance of a pentagonal resection of an eyelid margin tumour which may be close to the inferior lacrimal puntum (Fig 6.26a,b,c).

MOHS TECHNIQUE (Fig 6.27)

This is a frozen section technique which monitors the whole edge and base of a resected specimen. It is valuable when the tumour has ill-defined edges and depth extension such as may occur with a morphoeic BCC or with a recurrent tumour. The Mohs surgeon excises the specimen under local anaesthetic (Fig 6.27a) and then takes a thin

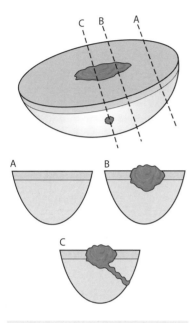

Figure 6.25

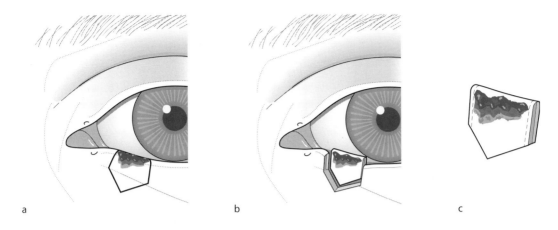

Figure 6.26

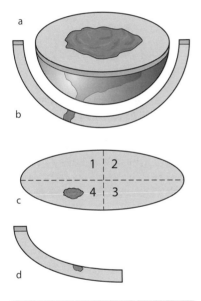

Figure 6.27

section of the whole edge and base of what has been resected (Fig 6.27b). This section is divided into four and the edges of each quarter section are colour coded. They are examined as frozen sections (Fig 6.27c). If there is any remaining tumour its site can be precisely identified and it can be excised until frozen sections of the edge and base are completely clear (Fig 6.27d). The patient is then ready for a definitive repair. The process is time consuming and requires special training but the results are excellent. Similar results can be obtained if urgent paraffin sections are used instead of frozen sections but the patient has to wait rather longer for repair of the wound.

If local tumour cannot be cleared without sacrificing the eye, an exenteration is indicated provided there is no evidence of distant spread.

DISTANT SPREAD

Malignant eyelid tumours such as malignant melanomas, meibomian gland or adenocarcinomas and squamous carcinomas may spread via the lymphatics or blood stream.

Lymphatic spread can be assessed by histological examination of the so-called 'sentinel node' or primary lymph node of the lymphatic drainage chain. A radioactive substance is injected close to the eyelid margin and a Geiger counter used to identify the relevant sentinel node which is usually in the preauricular or submandibular region. The site of the sentinel node is marked on the skin and the scintillogram recorded.

Prior to surgery later that day or the following day, an injection of a blue dye is made close to the tumour. This drains to the sentinel node which becomes blue. An excision biopsy is then carried out of the sentinel node which is identified at surgery firstly by the Geiger counter recording and secondly by its blue colour. In the preauricular region a nerve stimulator is used to identify and preserve the branches of the 7th nerve.

If the sentinel node does contain tumour the patient undergoes an appropriate block dissection of the relevant lymphatics.

Screening for distant spread of tumour other than to the lymphatics includes a general physical examination, chest x-ray to exclude pulmonary spread, liver function tests and body scans as appropriate. If distant spread occurs management usually involves an oncologist and various combinations of radiotherapy, chemotherapy, other drugs and immune system stimulation.

EXENTERATION

Principle

The globe is excised with all or part of the eyelids. The extent of the exenteration depends on which tissues are infiltrated with tumour.

Indications

Extensive tumour involvement of the ocular adnexae, which cannot be excised completely without removing the globe and surrounding tissues. If tumour involves the extraocular muscles it is unwise to try and save the eye except in special circumstances such as if it is the only seeing eye etc. Sometimes an exenteration is justified for 'toilet' reasons even if distant spread has occurred.

Method

1. Mark the area of the proposed excision. If the tumour is relatively posterior it may be possible to split the lids and save almost all of the lid skin. If the tumour involves only the upper lid, much of the lower lid skin can be saved.
2. Cut through the skin with a blade and extend the excision to the periosteum of the orbital rim with a cutting diathermy, if available.
3. Cut the periosteum of the orbital rim and raise it with an elevator to behind the globe.
4. The lacrimal sac must be mobilised and cut in the lacrimal fossa. Care must be taken with the thin lacrimal and medial orbital wall bones as a perforation may create a 'blow hole' connection with the nasal passages via the air cells.
5. Use curved blunt enucleation scissors to cut the mobilised periosteum and enclosed orbital contents as far behind the globe as required. This is governed by the position of the tumour, i.e. a choroidal malignant melanoma extending posteriorly will require as posterior an exenteration as possible.
6. Control the haemorrhage with local pressure for several minutes.
7. Reduce the skin defect as much as possible by suturing together whatever skin edges will close. If most of the skin of both lids

was saved, the socket can be completely lined, otherwise a variably sized bare area will be left.

8. Pack the socket with Vaseline gauze and a pressure dressing for 48 hours. If the skin edges were closed completely and a haematoma develops, this can be aspirated with a wide-bore needle and the pressure dressing reapplied.

9. Allow any open wound to granulate. Keep it clean with a simple antiseptic dressing such as chlorhexidine or half strength eusol and paraffin on a swab applied twice daily until the surface heals, leaving a smooth epithelialised socket. This may take 3 months or more if the open area was extensive. If it is not feasible to allow an open wound to granulate, the socket can be lined with a split skin graft.

ANTIMETABOLITES AND PHOTODYNAMIC TREATMENT

These forms of treatment are effective in certain instances but are beyond the scope of this book.

Repair of eyelid injuries

7

IMMEDIATE MANAGEMENT

1. *Examine and treat patient for all injuries.*
   Any eyelid injury may be part of more general trauma. A full ocular examination, including x-rays, CT, MRI and ultrasound, may be required as well as the exclusion of damage to the brain, skull, skeleton, thorax, abdomen, etc.

2. *Delay any repair until conditions are favourable.*
   The results of eyelid surgery are not prejudiced by waiting for up to 48 or 72 hours if this allows more time and better facilities to be made available.

3. *Remove all dirt and foreign bodies.*
   Every attempt should be made at the initial repair to clean the wound thoroughly to prevent subsequent tattooing, etc., and to remove all foreign bodies.

4. *Reposition the tissues as accurately as possible.*
   All wounds should be examined carefully and any visible damage repaired, but the wound should not be extended to explore structures that may not be damaged, e.g. the levator complex, unless the exploration is for a suspected foreign body.

5. *Do not excise or discard tissue.*
   The excellent blood supply in the eyelid region often allows tissue to survive as a free graft, but any pedicle should be preserved if possible. It is not usually necessary to cut or 'freshen' the wound edges.

6. *Delay major reconstruction.*
   Preferably do not add tissue at the primary repair unless the cornea is seriously at risk. It is better to wait for the wound to settle for 3, 6 or even 9 months before repairing a defect such as lid retraction, scars or ptosis unless the patient develops signs of corneal exposure that cannot easily be controlled with simple lubricants, etc.

LACRIMAL DRAINAGE INJURIES

IMMEDIATE INJURIES

UPPER CANALICULUS

It is rare to get symptoms from a blocked upper canaliculus if the lower canaliculus is functioning normally. It is therefore unreasonable to use any method to repair an upper canaliculus that might jeopardise the patency of the lower canaliculus.

LOWER CANALICULUS (Fig 7.1)

The repair of lower canaliculus injuries is controversial (Fig 7.1a). It is not difficult to suture together the two ends of a canaliculus, but it is less easy to ensure that the anastomosis remains patent after several months. Intubation and various stents have been used but the stents themselves may induce fibrosis. It is safe to marsupialise or open the lacerated medial canaliculus into the conjunctival sac, repair the eyelid accurately and ignore the lacrimal punctum and lateral canaliculus (Fig 7.1b). If the upper canaliculus is intact, it probably drains most of the tears and its patency will not be jeopardised by such a repair.

COMMON CANALICULUS

If the injury involves a common canaliculus, it must be repaired or opened into the lacrimal sac, the canaliculae intubated and a dacryocystorhinostomy performed.

LACRIMAL SAC

If the lacrimal sac is injured, a dacryocystorhinostomy must be performed.

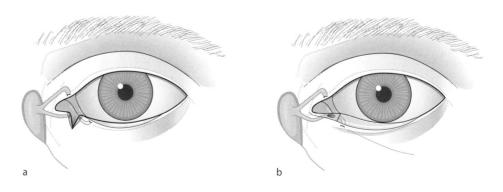

a   b

Figure 7.1

ESTABLISHED INJURIES

The management of established canalicular blockage depends on the position of blockage. If it is near the punctum it may be possible to open the lacrimal sac, retro-intubate a canaliculus and marsupialise it into the conjunctival sac. If the block is near the lacrimal sac, it may be possible to excise the scar and join the patent canaliculus to the sac. In either case it is necessary to have about 8 mm of one salvageable canaliculus for any effective functional drainage to occur. If the canaliculae are more extensively damaged, a lacrimal bypass procedure is required. If the lacrimal sac is opened it is wise to always perform a dacryocystorhinostomy. The management of other lacrimal drainage obstruction is covered in Chapter 8.

MEDIAL CANTHAL TENDON INJURIES AND TRAUMATIC TELECANTHUS

The principles governing the immediate management of medial canthal tendon injuries are the same as those for eyelid lacerations. The tissues must be repositioned as accurately as possible and any lacrimal drainage injury should be managed as described above. It is rarely necessary to repair the anterior limb of the medial canthal tendon only. The principal aim is to reform the posterior limb of the medial canthal tendon, and the technique depends on the posterior fixation point available.

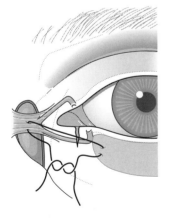

MEDIAL CANTHAL TENDON ANTERIOR LIMB RECONSTRUCTION (Fig 7.2)

Principle
A nonabsorbable or wire suture is used to reform the anterior limb of the medial canthal tendon.

Indications
Damage to the medial canthal tendon limited to its anterior limb. If the posterior limb of the medial canthal tendon is damaged at the same time and only the anterior limb is repaired, the lid will tend to be antero-positioned.

Figure 7.2

Method
1. If the injury is relatively lateral, see plication of anterior limb of medial canthal tendon (Fig 7.2; p 63).
2. If the injury is relatively medial, see medial canthal tendon shortening (p 157).

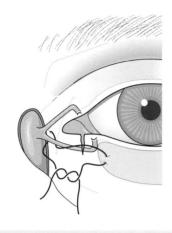

Figure 7.3

MEDIAL CANTHAL TENDON POSTERIOR LIMB RECONSTRUCTION

MEDIAL ORBITAL WALL FIXATION (Fig 7.3)

Principle

The medial eyelid tissues are attached to the medial orbital wall with a nonabsorbable or wire suture.

Indications

Telecanthus and damage to the posterior limb of the medial canthal tendon when the lacrimal drainage system is intact, provided that a firm and reasonably positioned medial orbital wall fixation point can be found.

Method

See plication of posterior limb of medial canthal tendon (Fig 7.3; p 64) and medial canthal resection (p 67).

POSTLACRIMAL SAC FIXATION (Fig 7.4)

Principle

A nonabsorbable or wire suture is passed behind the open lacrimal sac and used to reattach the medial canthal and eyelid tissues medially and posteriorly to the posterior lacrimal sac fascia.

Indications

Telecanthus and damage to the posterior limb of the medial canthal tendon, when the lacrimal sac must be opened for a dacryocystorhinostomy provided that the tissues behind the lacrimal sac are adequate. If they are not adequate a firm posterior fixation must be obtained with a bone screw and suture, mini plate to which a suture can be attached, or transnasal wire.

Method

1. After carrying out stages 1–3 of a DCR (p 169), push a curved 25 mm or larger needle with a nonabsorbable or wire suture through the periosteal tissues behind the fundus of the opened lacrimal sac, and retrieve it from the nose (Fig 7.4a).
2. Pass the needle back approximately parallel to its original course (Fig 7.4b).
3. Pick up the tarsus or whatever medial canthal structures are available and tie the suture (Fig 7.4c,d).
   Note: a. The suture can be attached to the medial canthal structures or tarsus and both arms of the suture then passed behind the lacrimal sac so that it is tied in the nose. The

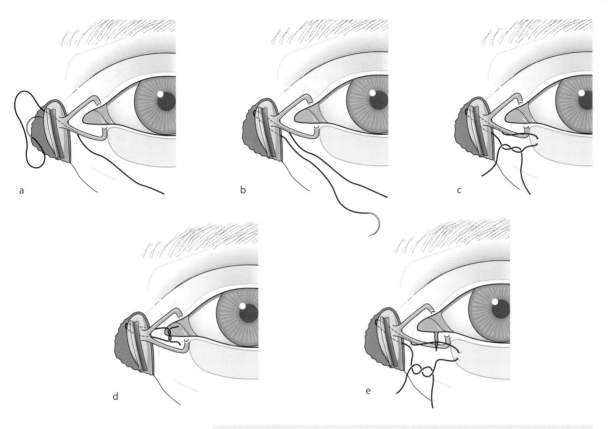

Figure 7.4

knot will be buried when the posterior flaps of lacrimal and nasal mucosa are sutured.

b. Any canalicular damage must be managed as previously described (Fig 7.4e)

4. Complete the DCR stages 14–18 (p 171).

TRANSNASAL WIRE (Figs 7.5, 7.6)

Principle

A wire is passed across the nose and attached to the medial canthal tissues on each side. When it is tightened the intercanthal distance is reduced. It may be necessary to remove bone and scar tissue to get an adequate correction. A DCR is usually necessary and the wire is then passed through the wall of the opened lacrimal sac (Fig 7.5a), but this is not always required (Fig 7.5b) (see p 157). The wire may be attached directly to the medial canthal structures (Fig 7.5a,b) or indirectly to the tarsus (Fig 7.5c).

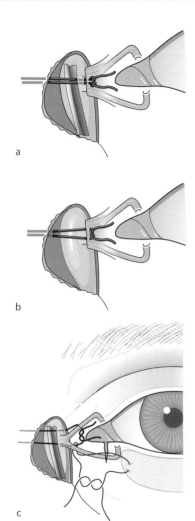

a

b

c

Figure 7.5

Indications

Telecanthus, when no adequate ipsilateral posterior fixation point can be found. A bone screw and suture can be used as an alternative but depends on adequate bone being available exactly where the posterior fixation is required. Another option is a mini plate which can be screwed to firm bone with an extension to the desired posterior fixation point to which a suture can be attached. A transnasal wire does not depend on an attachment to bone and is therefore usually the best technique after trauma when a wide clearance of fractured bone and scar is often required to allow correction of traumatic telecanthus.

Method

1. Expose the medial canthal structures with a Y-shaped incision or whatever is appropriate in the particular circumstances (see Fig 7.9a)
2. Try to identify what remains of the lacrimal fossa, incise the periosteum over it and reflect it laterally with the lacrimal sac.
3. Remove all excess bone with, for example, a hammer and chisel, burr or bone-nibbling forceps, and excise and free adhesions and scar tissue until the medial canthus can be correctly positioned.
4. Treat the lacrimal drainage system as indicated. Usually this involves carrying out a DCR and closing the posterior lacrimal sac and nasal mucosal flaps as appropriate — stages 1–4 (p 169).
5. Expose the medial canthal tendon on the contralateral side.
6. Leave the medial canthal attachment of the tendon intact and cut the periosteum over the anterior lacrimal crest.
7. Elevate the periosteum over the lacrimal fossa and reflect it laterally with the lacrimal sac.
8. Pass a curved needle under the medial canthal tendon close to its periosteal attachment, avoiding damage to the lacrimal sac, and pull a loop of wire around the tendon (Fig 7.6a).
9. Pass both ends of this wire through the eye of a Mustardé awl or a Wright's fascial needle with a 4 '0' nylon suture and introduce the instrument into the lacrimal fossa as far posterior as possible (Fig 7.6b).
10. Push the instrument across the nose into the rhinostomy or lacrimal fossa area (Fig 7.6c). Remove both ends of the wire and the nylon suture before inserting another nylon suture through the eye and withdrawing the instrument.
11. Fix the two ends of the wire directly (Fig 7.6d) or indirectly (see Fig 7.12c) to whatever firm medial canthal structures are available. If the lacrimal sac is open the wire will pass through the dacryocystorhinostomy (see Fig 7.5a), but it can be passed anterior to an intact lacrimal sac (see Fig 7.5b).
12. Twist the wire to correct the telecanthus as required and bury the ends of the wire (Fig 7.6e).
13. Close the anterior lacrimal sac and nasal mucosal flaps as appropriate.

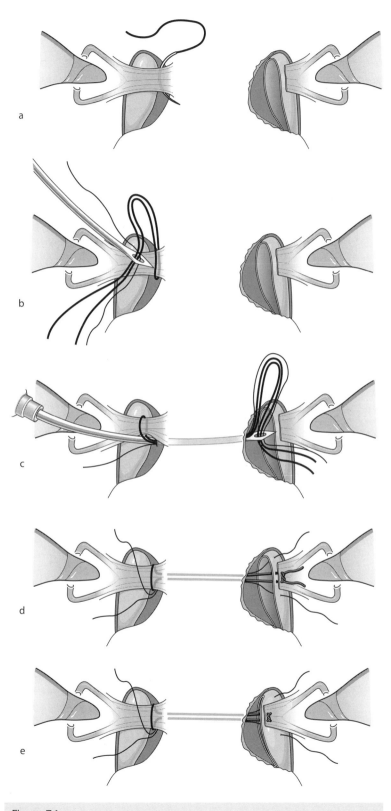

Figure 7.6

14. Pass the nylon sutures through the skin on either side of the wounds. Suture the skin edges and tie the nylon sutures over bolsters which can be removed after 3–5 days (see Fig 7.12e).

Complications

With any medial canthal tendon reconstruction there is a tendency for recurrence of the eyelid malposition and telecanthus. At surgery the deformity should therefore always be overcorrected. Nonabsorbable sutures can lead to granulomas etc.

CORRECTION OF EPICANTHIC FOLDS AND TELECANTHUS

Epicanthic folds may be congenital or acquired as a result of trauma. They are caused by a shortage of skin. The treatment is to lengthen the fold with a Z-plasty or double Z-plasty and to excise any scar tissue if appropriate. The Z-plasty can be combined with medial canthal tendon and lacrimal surgery if necessary. If medial canthal tendon shortening and telecanthus correction is required without surgery to an epicanthic fold, a Y-V plasty approach is useful. If an epicanthic fold needs to be corrected at the same time as a medial canthal tendon shortening, a Z-plasty or double Z-plasty is combined with a Y-V plasty as in the Mustardé technique. If there is an increase in the bony intercanthal distance (hyperteleorism) as opposed to an increase in the soft tissue intercanthal distance (telecanthus), bone must be removed and the intercanthal distance reduced by wiring the two medial canthi together with a trans-nasal wire. These techniques can be applied equally to the correction of trauma or other conditions such as the blepharophimosis syndrome.

EPICANTHIC Z-PLASTY (Fig 7.7)

Principle

Two flaps of skin are transposed to change the line of a fold and lengthen it (see Fig 4.15a)

Indications

A simple epicanthic fold.

Method

1. Mark the central limb of the Z in the line of the fold.
2. Draw the other two limbs approximately the same length. The shape of the Z and the angle between the limbs depend on the space available (Fig 7.7a).
3. Raise the flaps, excise any scar tissue, transpose them and suture the skin edges (Fig 7.7b).

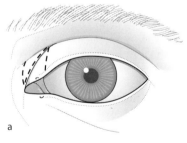

a

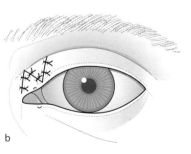

b

Figure 7.7

DOUBLE Z-PLASTY (SPAETH) (Fig 7.8)

Principle

A separate Z-plasty is used to lengthen and change the position of a fold affecting both upper and lower eyelids.

Indications

An epicanthic fold involving both lids without telecanthus (Fig 7.8a).

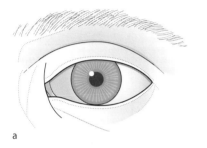
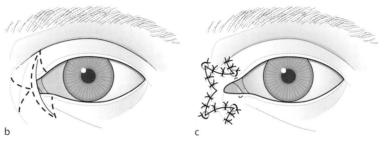

a   b   c

Figure 7.8

Method

1. Mark a Z on each lid with two of the apices joining over the medial canthal tendon (Fig 7.8b).
2. Raise and transpose the flaps (Fig 7.8c).

Y-V MEDIAL CANTHOPLASTY (Fig 7.9)

Principle

A horizontal Y-shaped incision is made over the medial canthal tendon which can be shortened to correct any telecanthus. The Y-shaped incision is then sutured as a V.

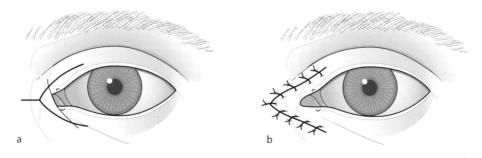

a   b

Figure 7.9

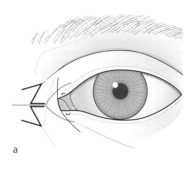

a

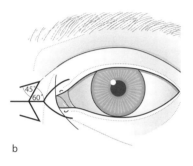

b

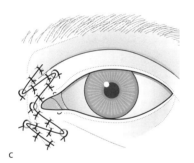

c

Figure 7.10

Indications

Exposure of medial canthal tendon for correction of telecanthus if there is no significant associated epicanthus. It allows correction of the telecanthus associated with the blepharophimosis syndrome and gives good access for the repair of medial canthal tendon injuries with a DCR if necessary.

Method

1. Mark a Y on the medial canthal skin with the base of the stem in the desired new position of the medial canthus (Fig 7.9a).
2. Cut the flaps and trim them.
3. Excise excess subcutaneous tissue in the blepharophimosis syndrome or post-traumatic scar tissue and shorten the medial canthal tendon if required.
4. Use buried 6 '0' long-acting absorbable sutures to fix the subcutaneous tissues to the medial canthal tendon. Close the skin as a V with fine absorbable sutures which can be removed in an adult (Fig 7.9b).

   Note: if much subcutaneous tissue has been excised, the reformed canthus will be relatively posterior and the wound can only be closed as a Y shape.

DOUBLE Z-PLASTY (MUSTARDÉ) (Fig 7.10)

Principle

A double Z and a Y-V plasty are combined (Fig 7.10a). The double Z lengthens and changes the position of the epicanthic fold, and the Y-V plasty, with shortening of the medial canthal tendon, corrects the telecanthus.

Indications

A marked epicanthic fold associated with telecanthus, especially if there is an entropion caused by traction from the fold. This is mainly relevant to correction of the blepharophimosis syndrome.

Method

1. Make a mark on the skin at the site of the present medial canthus and at the site of the proposed medial canthus.
2. Join these lines and from the centre draw two lines extending laterally at an angle of approximately 60°. These form the main limbs of the Z-plasty.
3. From the end of each limb draw a nearly horizontal line which angles slightly towards the proposed new medial canthus at approximately 45° to the main limb of the Z.
4. Draw a line laterally from the present medial canthus close to the upper and lower lid margin. This completes the skin marks in the figure of a 'flying man' (Fig 7.10b).

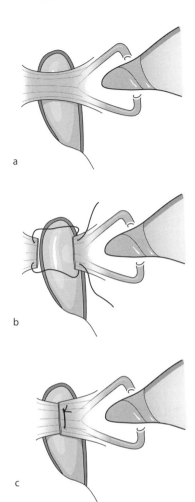

a

b

c

Figure 7.11

5. Cut through the skin along these marks.
6. Excise the underlying subcutaneous tissue and muscle until the medial canthal tendon is exposed. In the blepharophimosis syndrome the tendon is usually elongated, thin and buried under abnormal tissue.
7. Shorten the medial canthal tendon if required.
8. Suture the subcutaneous tissues in the region of the old medial canthus to the subcutaneous and deep tissues in the region of the new medial canthus.
9. Transpose the skin flaps.
10. Suture the skin flaps with 6 '0' nylon, or 6 '0' long-acting absorbable sutures in a child (Fig 7.10c).
11. Apply local pressure dressings for 2 days if possible but leave the eyes open.

MEDIAL CANTHAL TENDON SHORTENING WITH CANTHOPLASTY (Fig 7.11)

Principle

The medial canthal tendon is exposed and shortened with a non-absorbable or wire suture (Fig 7.11).

Indications

Telecanthus, often associated with the blepharophimosis syndrome. Post-traumatic medial canthal tendon repair usually involves associated injury to the lacrimal drainage apparatus and is described above.

Method

1. Expose the medial canthal tendon (Fig 7.11a). Use a Y-V plasty if there is no epicanthic fold and a double Z plasty if there is a significant epicanthic fold.
2. Place a probe in the inferior canaliculus.
3. Free the tendon from the underlying lacrimal sac tissues.
4. Resect the middle portion of the tendon (Fig 7.11b).
5. Suture the lateral portion of the tendon to the periosteum and medial stump of the tendon with a nonabsorbable or wire suture (Fig 7.11c).
6. Close the skin wound.

MEDIAL CANTHAL TENDON SHORTENING WITH TRANSNASAL WIRE (Fig 7.12)

Principle

The intercanthal distance is reduced by removing bone and wiring the two medial canthal tendons together across the nose.

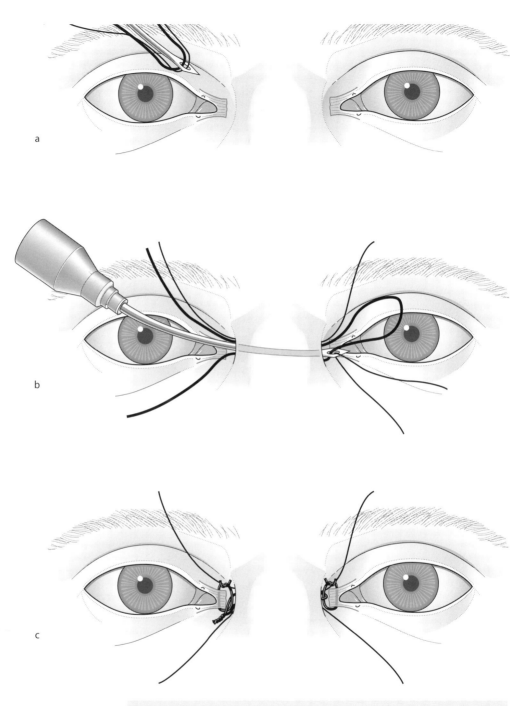

Figure 7.12

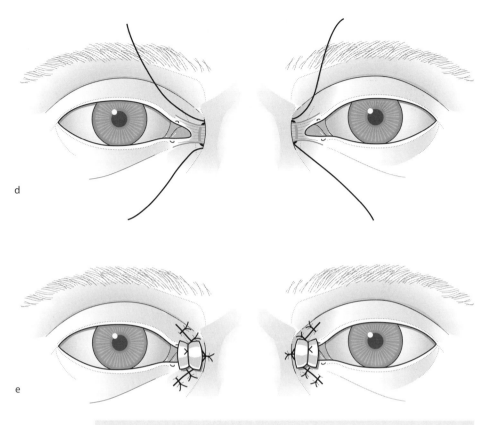

d

e

Figure 7.12 cont'd

Indications

Severe telecanthus and hypertelorism, e.g. associated with the blepharophimosis syndrome when bone must be removed bilaterally to reduce the intercanthal distance (it is not usually necessary to do a DCR); after major medial canthal tumour surgery, etc; for trauma see p 148.

Method

1. Expose and resect the medial canthal tendons as described above for medial canthal tendon shortening with canthoplasty.
2. Reduce the bone of the anterior lacrimal crest and reflect the lacrimal sac laterally. Follow method for transnasal wire for traumatic telecanthus (p 151).
3. Pass a Mustardé awl across the nose with a wire and a 4 '0' nylon suture (Fig 7.12a).

4. Leave a loop of wire across the nose and one 4 '0' nylon suture (Fig 7.12b).
5. Withdraw the awl with another 4 '0' nylon suture and the end of the wire leaving the loop behind.
6. Suture the resected medial canthal tendons to the transnasal wire loop (Fig 7.12c).
7. Twist the wire to tighten it and correct the telecanthus (Fig 7.12d).
8. Pass the 4 '0' nylon sutures through the medial canthoplasty flaps. Tie them together over bolsters to keep pressure on the wound (Fig 7.12e).
9. Remove the sutures after 5 days.

Complications

Scarring. This is the risk with all small flaps used for medial cantho-plasties. It can be minimised with pressure vibromassage, steroid creams etc. There is a tendency for relapse of any correction of tele-canthus and hypertelorism. The deformity should be overcorrected at the time of surgery. Massage may increase the risk of relapse. There are the usual risks of granulomas and exposure with permanent and wire sutures. Any surgery around the lacrimal drainage apparatus can cause epiphora.

ORBITAL FRACTURES

ORBITAL FLOOR AND MEDIAL WALL FRACTURES

DIAGNOSIS

The orbital floor and medial wall is relatively easily fractured. The diagnosis depends on a high index of clinical suspicion and signs of diplopia (usually vertical) plus hypoaesthesia in the maxillary division of the 5th nerve. The diagnosis should be confirmed with x-rays including preferably CT and MRI scans. The patients should be given systemic antibiotics since the fractures are compound into the sinuses.

INDICATIONS FOR SURGERY

The initial management depends on the degree of enophthalmos, size of fracture and whether there is vertical diplopia with radiolog-ical evidence of entrapment of muscles, particularly the inferior rec-tus muscle. If there is more than 3 mm of enophthalmos within the first 10 days, a large fracture site or entrapped muscles with diplopia which is not improving, the fracture site should be explored via a lateral canthal or anterior approach (p 214), the defect repaired or the entrapped muscle released. Sometimes it is difficult to decide on the clinical significance of the radiological evidence of apparent muscle entrapment. In these cases the diplopia must be carefully monitored and if it is not improving after 10 days it is wise to explore the socket.

Method

Follow lateral canthal or anterior approach to orbital floor (p 214, see Figs 11.8, 11.9). If the orbit is explored it is usually reasonable to repair the fracture with a thin silastic sheet inserted subperiosteally and held in position by re-suturing the periosteum. If the fracture site is large or there is a possibility of infection an autogenous bone graft is preferable. If there is a significant volume deficit and hypotropia which is not adequately corrected by elevating the fracture, the orbital floor implant should be increased in size but not so much that the globe is elevated above the level of the contra lateral eye.

The vision and pupillary reactions should be checked in the recovery room immediately after the surgery has finished and over the next 12–18 hours. If there is any evidence of pupillary dilatation or decreased vision it may be necessary to remove the implant as an emergency.

Complications

Loss of vision, diplopia, enophthalmos, infection, implant extrusion etc as described under orbital floor implants (p 214).

COMMINUTED ORBITAL RIM FRACTURES

These usually require direct exposure and fixation.

ZYGOMATIC FRACTURES

These can usually be corrected with an elevator placed under the zygomatic arch via a temporal incision in the hair line.

ORBITAL ROOF FRACTURES

These should be managed with a neurosurgeon.

TRAUMATIC PTOSIS

Wounds involving the levator complex should be managed as for any eyelid injury. Every attempt should be made at the primary repair to reposition the various tissue layers as accurately as possible and to remove all foreign bodies. The lacerations should not be routinely extended to examine the levator complex away from the wound unless the levator has been very obviously transected and the two ends cannot be identified. After the initial repair of the wound, if there is a residual ptosis the lid should be left alone for 6 months or longer while there are continuing signs of improvement. It should then be explored, preferably under local anaesthesia, via the anterior approach (p 96 and 100). If the surgery is carried out under general anaesthesia, adjustable sutures may be helpful (p 107, Fig 5.9).

A traumatic ptosis can be caused by the following, either separately or in combination: a direct injury or stretching of the aponeurosis; a direct injury or bruising of the levator muscle; a lowering of the fulcrum of the levator complex which is normally provided by the globe and Whitnall's ligament, e.g. a phthisical eye, loss of orbital contents from orbital wall fractures, surgery etc; an injury to the third or sympathetic nerve supply anywhere in its course to the levator and Müller's muscle; or a mechanical restriction which can occur as a conjunctival symblepharon or scar, or deep within the lid and orbit.

The cause of the ptosis is often not obvious and therefore after 6 months if there are no further signs of recovery, the lid should be explored as described above and an attempt made to advance the levator complex. If this is contraindicated because of the cause, appropriate treatment should be instigated e.g. for a 3rd nerve palsy (see p 89). If the upper lid is explored and scar tissue is excised this may leave a gap in the levator complex which, if repaired directly, would cause lid retraction. It is wise to have a 'spacer' such as ear cartilage, Alloderm or sclera available in case this occurs. If there are dense adhesions it may be possible to reduce their tendency to reform by interposing a dermis fat graft as described for upper lid sulcus reconstruction on p 217. A defective skin crease without a ptosis can be reformed as described on p 106. If a proper attempt has been made to find and shorten the upper lid retractor complex and the ptosis remains with no significant lid movement, the lid should be elevated with a frontalis sling/brow suspension procedure provided there are no contraindications e.g. absent frontalis muscle action, limited ocular movements etc.

CORNEAL EXPOSURE, SCARS AND TISSUE LOSS

If the immediate repair of an eyelid laceration has been reasonably well performed, it is wise to wait until any scars or defects are quiescent before considering further treatment unless corneal exposure occurs that cannot be controlled with simple lubricants, etc.

CORNEAL EXPOSURE

Corneal exposure following trauma may be caused by the following, either separately or in combination:

- Anterior (p 115) or posterior (p 117) lamella defects and scar.
  – Treatment. Localised: Z-plasty. Generalised: graft or flap.
- Full-thickness lid defects (p 122)

– Treatment. The choice of repair in any individual case is governed by the position of the scars.
- Scarring of lid retractors.
  – Treatment. Upper lid: retractor recession procedure (p 196). Lower lid: retractor lengthening (p 200).
- 7th nerve palsy (p 177)
  – Treatment. Reduce palpebral aperture, improve eyelid closure
- Restricted ocular movements from adhesions or nerve palsies
  – Treatment. Free adhesions, reduce palpebral aperture.
- Reduced tear film.
  – Treatment. Lubricants, reduce palpebral aperture etc.

SCAR REVISION (Fig 7.13)

Principle

The aims of scar revision are the excision of all scar and fibrous tissue, careful, accurate realignment of tissues, and the break-up and alteration of the line of the wound so that when fibrosis occurs the contraction is not in the same line as previously and the scar is less obvious if it is irregular. Ideally the scar should be altered to be hidden in a natural fold or crease.

Indications

Symptoms of corneal exposure; a mature unsightly scar. A scar can be considered mature when it is no longer red. This may take 6 months or much longer.

Method

A mature scar can be excised and carefully resutured but it is better to break up the line of the scar with a Z-plasty (p 73) (Fig 7.13a) or preferably a double (Fig 7.13b) or multiple Z-plasty. This breaks up the line of the scar better and reduces the tension at the apices of individual flaps by spreading it over a greater number of smaller flaps. Postoperative management with pressure vibromassage and local steroids is often very helpful.

TRAUMATIC AVULSION OF BOTH EYELIDS

Principle

The conjunctival remnants from the fornices and globe are sutured together over the cornea and covered with a split skin graft.

Indications

Total eyelid loss with retention of the globe, e.g. degloving injury.

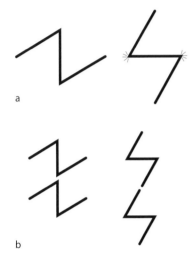

a

b

Figure 7.13

Method

1. Explore the conjunctival fornices and free any conjunctival elements that have been pulled behind the orbital rim by the lid retractors.

2. Dissect the conjunctiva from the lid retractors and from the globe if necessary until it can be pulled together over the cornea and closed with fine interrupted absorbable sutures.

3. Cover the raw surface of the conjunctiva and the globe if necessary with a split skin graft. It should be possible to cover the orbital rim with skin flaps but, if necessary, a split skin graft will take on this exposed bone provided that any relatively avascular outer table of bone is removed.

4. After many months an attempt can be made to open the split skin and conjunctiva in front of the eye, but there is a marked tendency for the flaps to contract, and extensive repeated reconstructive surgery is usually required.

Lacrimal surgery

8

Tears are essential for the normal function of the eye. Those tears not lost by evaporation drain to the inferior meatus of the nose via the membranous tear passages. The volume of tears being produced at any particular moment is controlled by the lacrimal nucleus of the parasympathetic nervous system, the activity of which is largely determined reflexly by the fifth cranial nerve. If this volume exceeds the normal drainage capacity of the system, or if the passages are obstructed, then inevitably tears will spill onto the cheek to give rise to the troublesome symptom of epiphora. Watering that can be attributed to overproduction of tears (lacrimation) usually responds to medical measures directed to the treatment of its cause (e.g. blepharitis). Watering caused by an obstruction (obstructive epiphora) can nearly always be relieved by surgery. The type of procedure applicable is determined by the aetiology and level of the obstruction in the system.

In addition to epiphora, a patient with lacrimal obstruction may also be troubled by the presence of a mucocele with its attendant mucous or mucopurulent discharge. The overfull tear film interferes with vision and, occasionally, invasion of the obstructed tear passages by pyogenic organisms gives rise to a painful attack of acute dacryocystitis. If the obstruction is not relieved, this may itself be complicated by fistula formation. Obstruction in the tear passages represents a hazard when intraocular surgery is to be performed.

Although recent advances in instrumentation have allowed lacrimal drainage surgery to be performed endoscopically either through the nose or via the canaliculae, the results are as yet not as good as those obtained with the classical skin approach which is described here. The endoscopic approach does allow the surgery to be performed without creating any skin incision and scar. A DCR skin incision however usually heals very well and does not create a significant cosmetic blemish.

ASSESSMENT OF LACRIMAL SYSTEM

HISTORY

A carefully elicited history will frequently provide clues as to the diagnosis, e.g.:

- Red eye, blisters on lid: herpetic canalicular obstruction
- Persistent watering and discharge despite repeated patent syringing: *Streptothrix* infection
- Previous surgery: ?dacryocystectomy.

EXAMINATION

Purpose: to decide whether the patient is lacrimating or has an obstructive cause for their symptoms and, if it is an obstruction, to accurately define its level. Obstruction can have a functional or anatomical basis.

1. Lids: lid laxity, facial weakness, lacrimal fistulae, blepharitis, tarsal scarring, etc.
2. Globe and bulbar conjunctiva: conjunctival scarring, e.g. trachoma; intraocular pathology, e.g. sarcoid, syphilis.
3. Tear passages:
   a. Tests to determine the anatomical state of the passages.
      (i) *Syringing.* Having dilated the punctum, insert the tip of a lacrimal cannula into the ampulla at right angles to the lid margin. Draw the lid laterally and rotate the tip of the cannula medially, advancing its tip some 4–5 mm along the canaliculus. Gently irrigate with saline. If fluid regurgitates along the opposite canaliculus, this confirms patency at least as far as the common canaliculus. Should fluid flow back along the same canaliculus, then the tip of the cannula can be advanced to try and identify the position of the block. If mucus regurgitates, this usually implies a blockage located within the sac or the nasolacrimal duct. The cannula may be introduced into the lacrimal sac but great care must be exercised as it is easy to create artefactual passages or to damage the valves around the internal common opening. The passage of saline to the nasopharynx confirms the patency but not the normality of the tear passages.
      (ii) *Diagnostic probing.* Use Liebrich's 0 or 00 probe to identify the level of any canalicular blockage, fistula tracts, etc.
      (iii) *Dacryocystography.* Identify the level of obstruction, tumours, stenosis, diverticulae, fistulae, *Streptothrix* organisms, etc.
      (iv) *Nasal examination.* Exclude nasal disease, rhinitis, polyps, deviated septum, turbinates, etc.
   b. Tests to demonstrate the functional state of the tear passages. The object of these tests is to monitor the progress through the tear passages of substances introduced into the conjunctival sac.
      (i) *Dye tests.* A coloured fluid such as 2% fluorescein or 10% protargolum is introduced into the conjunctival sac. A cotton wool tipped swab is introduced along the

interior meatus of the nose some 30 mm to the lower end of the nasolacrimal duct, and if the dye can be recovered after 2 minutes the test is said to be positive. If no dye is recovered then the dye is washed from the conjunctival sac and the system syringed with saline. If dye now appears in the nose, this is referred to as a positive secondary dye test.

(ii) *Taste tests*. Substances whose arrival in the nasopharynx can be recognised by their taste, such as saccharine or picric acid, may be utilised.

(iii) *Lacrimal scintillography*. A qualitative and quantitative assessment of lacrimal drainage function can be made using a suitably modified gamma-camera to monitor the progress of radioactively labelled tears through the system. Negative results to any of the above tests should be interpreted with great caution and never without having studied properly executed dacryocystograms.

MANAGEMENT OF LACRIMAL OBSTRUCTION

CONGENITAL NASOLACRIMAL DUCT OBSTRUCTION

This is present in some 6% of newborn babies. Spontaneous resolution without surgical intervention can be anticipated in the majority of cases by the age of 1 year. It is reasonable therefore to adopt an expectant regimen of management certainly for several months, unless an attack of acute dacryocystitis intervenes. The mother is instructed on the importance of lid hygiene and asked to instil some antibiotic drops or ointment such as Chloromycetin on a regular basis.

Between the ages of 6 and 9 months, should the symptoms persist, an examination should be carried out under an anaesthetic. In the event of acute dacryocystitis, systemic antibiotics should be administered for 24 hours before the examination. Dilate a punctum and introduce the tip of a lacrimal cannula into the tear sac, being careful to obtain a 'hard stop' (i.e. that the tip of the cannula has reached the medial sac wall) before rotating the cannula downwards to enter the body of the sac. If patency is not obtained on gentle syringing, the tip of the cannula, or that of a fine lacrimal probe inserted to replace it, is advanced down the medial sac wall to enter the nasolacrimal duct which is gently probed. Whether one carries out the manipulations using the upper or lower canaliculus is of little importance provided that care is exercised. The common canaliculus is vulnerable to injury by either route. That patency has been achieved can be confirmed by observing the presence of saline in the nose following a further syringing. If the nasolacrimal duct cannot be probed, then it is possible that there is a bony abnormality present and the procedure should be aborted. Local antibiotics are prescribed for 3 weeks following the probing. In the event of the procedure not having brought about a resolution of the symptoms, then it can be repeated after about 3 months. On this second occasion it may well be helpful to obtain a dacryocystogram to define the level of the sac obstruction.

If two technically satisfactory syringing and probing procedures have been carried out and symptoms persist, the canaliculae and nasolacrimal duct can be intubated. Various specially designed probes and tubes are available. The simplest is fine tubing with a malleable probe attached to each end. One probe is passed through the upper or lower canaliculus and retrieved from below the inferior turbinate. A grooved director can be placed under the inferior turbinate to help guide the probe out through the nostril. The other probe is then passed the same way through the other canaliculus. The tubes are tied in the nose and left for a minimum of 6 months or longer. It is important not to tie the tubes too tightly or they can cut through the lacrimal puncta and canaliculae. They are removed by simply cutting the loop of tubing at the medial canthus and pulling the tubes out through the nose.

If symptoms recur or it was not possible to probe the nasolacrimal duct a dacryocystorhinostomy is required to cure the child's condition. This operation is most conveniently performed at the age of 3–4 years, before attendance at school. Earlier intervention may be necessary in the presence of recurrent dacryocystitis. Some surgeons are not happy with intubating the lacrimal drainage system as there is a morbidity to the canaliculae from the introduction and presence of the tubing. If it was not possible to probe the nasolacrimal duct or if symptoms persisted despite two technically satisfactory syringing and probing procedures, they would wait until the child was 3–4 years old and then proceed directly with a dacryocystorhinostomy, if the condition had not cured itself spontaneously.

INDICATIONS FOR LACRIMAL DRAINAGE SURGERY

A blocked nasolacrimal drainage system causing epiphora; visual impairment from an over full tear film or discharge in the tear film; pain from acute dacryocystitis or an acute blockage of the lacrimal drainage system e.g. with a stone; discharge from chronic dacryocystitis and a mucocele or streptothrix infection, especially if intraocular surgery is proposed; fistula either congenital or acquired from acute dacryocystitis or trauma; trauma or neoplasm obstructing the nasolacrimal drainage system.

ANAESTHESIA

Lacrimal surgery can be carried out conveniently using general or local anaesthesia. General anaesthesia has the advantage that both the airway and blood pressure can be controlled. If a local anaesthetic is preferred, spray the nostril with an anaesthetic and vasoconstrictor solution such as cocaine 4% to which a drop of 1:1000 epinephrine has been added. Apply some 30% cocaine paste to the tip of a dressed orange stick and place it on the lateral wall of the nose adjacent to the tear sac.

Infiltrate the skin over the tear sac with xylocaine 2% with dilute epinephrine. Block the nasociliary nerve around the anterior ethmoidal foramen by introducing the needle just below the trochlea. As the needle is withdrawn, the tissue around the fundus of the sac is infiltrated. The needle is then directed to infiltrate the tissue along the anterior lacrimal crest and around the nasolacrimal duct. The superior alveolar nerve can be blocked as it leaves the infraorbital nerve to enter an osseous canal proximal to the infraorbital foramen.

DACRYOCYSTORHINOSTOMY (Fig 8.1)

Principle

The bone lying between the tear sac and the nose is removed and that part of the lacrimal sac that harbours the internal opening of the lacrimal canaliculi is incorporated into the lateral wall of the nose.

Indications

Any obstruction of the tear sac or nasolacrimal duct lying distal to the internal opening of the common canaliculus.

Method

1. Make a straight skin incision some 8 mm medial to the inner canthus. This should extend downwards and slightly laterally from a point some 2 mm above the lower border of the superficial part of the medial palpebral tendon for about 20 mm (Fig. 8.1a).

2. Separate the skin edges with 2 '0' silk traction sutures and identify the superficial part of the medial canthal tendon, being careful not to damage the angular vein that lies on the orbital part of the orbicularis.

3. Separate the orbital and palpebral fibres of the orbicularis to identify the periosteum over the orbital rim. Insert two or three traction sutures around the orbital orbicularis and attach them to the towels.

4. Divide the superficial part of the medial palpebral tendon and the periosteum just anterior to the orbital margin as far as a small spine on the anterior lacrimal crest, which usually lies in front of the exit of the nasolacrimal duct.

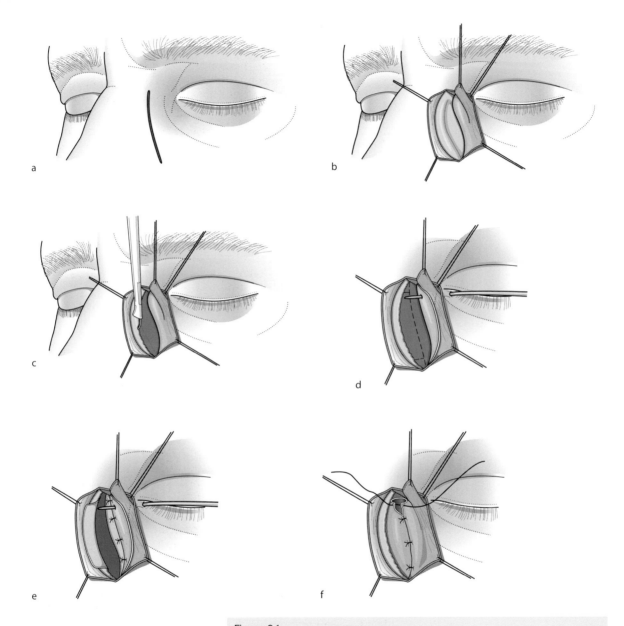

Figure 8.1

5. Use a periosteal elevator to reflect the periosteum forwards for some 5–7 mm and secure it with traction sutures.
6. Reflect the sac laterally from the floor of the fossa as far posterior as the posterior lacrimal crest to expose the whole floor of the fossa (Fig. 8.1b).
7. Separate the suture between the lacrimal bone and the frontal process of the maxilla, or that between the ethmoid and lacrimal bone, using an instrument such as the Traquair's periosteal elevator.

Note: should it prove impossible to make an opening into the nose with a periosteal elevator, the opening can be initiated using a bone trephine, drill or hammer and chisel.

8. Detach the nasal mucosa with the Traquair's elevator from the nasal aspect of the floor of the fossa and enlarge the opening with bone punches (Fig. 8.1c). Following each bite, reinsert the periosteal elevator to ensure that the nasal mucosa is separated from the bony margin of the developing rhinostomy, and not accidentally traumatised. When completed, the rhinostomy should extend from the top of the fossa, some 5 mm above the internal opening of the common canaliculus, downwards to include the first 5 mm of the bony nasolacrimal duct. The posterior margin should lie just anterior to the posterior lacrimal crest and should extend forward to include the whole of the floor of the fossa. The anterior lacrimal crest is removed, as is also that part of the frontal process of the maxilla that lies some 3–4 mm in front of the orbital margin.

Note: in the event of an anterior ethmoid air cell or the bony skeleton of the middle turbinate encroaching on the floor of the fossa, these may be removed.

9. Identify the sac lumen by passing a probe into it via a canaliculus.
10. Incise the medial wall of the sac vertically using a sac knife or a no. 11 blade and, using scissors, extend the incision upwards to the fundus of the sac and downwards into the nasolacrimal duct. The anterior and posterior flaps should be of equal size and should open like the leaves of a book.
11. Examine the internal common opening of the canaliculi and confirm its normality.
12. Make a vertical cut in the nasal mucosa, dividing it into an anterior two-thirds and a posterior one-third (Fig. 8.1d). Short horizontal relieving incisions may be necessary at the top and bottom of the anterior flap to allow it to swing forwards.
13. Pass a sucker up the nose and position its tip to lie just behind the posterior nasal mucosal flap.
14. Secure the posterior sac mucosal flap to that of the nose, using three or four interrupted 6 '0' long-acting absorbable sutures (Fig. 8.1e). This is most easily achieved in a backhand fashion from sac to nasal mucosa.

Note: the placement of posterior flap sutures is not universally undertaken. Their insertion, however, controls haemorrhage from that source, the mucosa-to-mucosa anastomosis precludes the development of granulation tissue with its possible attendant infection and secondary haemorrhage, and the fixation of the tissues in their desired position obviates the chance adhesion between the anterior and posterior flaps.

15. Approximate the anterior mucosal flaps with similar absorbable sutures, leaving the canalicular probe in position until the anastomosis is completed (Fig. 8.1f).

16. Reattach the divided superficial part of the medial palpebral tendon with a long-acting absorbable suture.
17. Close the skin with fine interrupted nylon sutures. Subcutaneous sutures are seldom necessary if the dissection has been carried out in the plane between the palpebral and orbital parts of the orbicularis muscle, and their presence can contribute to a prominent or lumpy scar.
18. Remove the sutures after 5 days. Postoperative antibiotics are unnecessary except in the presence of acute dacryocystitis but it is sensible to give a peroperative antibiotic cover.

Complications

Haemorrhage. If there is a problem at the time of surgery the area of the anastomosis between the nasal mucosal and lacrimal sac can be packed under direct vision and the pack removed after 12 hours. The incidence of postoperative haemorrhage is reduced if patients undergoing DCR are routinely given systemic antibiotics peroperatively. If haemorrhage does occur postoperatively and does not stop with simple measures such as sedation and holding the nose keeping the mouth open over a basin to collect the blood, the nose can be packed. Very occasionally a patient may need to be taken back to the operating theatre and the bleeding vessels identified and cauterised.

Recurrence of epiphora. Examine the patient as described above. The anastomosis should be inspected with an endoscope. Divide any adhesions and scar tissue and intubate the system. If this fails the DCR needs to be repeated or a CDCR or lacrimal bypass surgery performed as appropriate.

CANALICULAR OBSTRUCTIONS

THE COMMON CANALICULUS

Medial or membranous obstruction

The common canaliculus may become obstructed at its junction with the lumen of the sac as a complication of chronic dacryocystitis. This accounts for about two-thirds of common canaliculus obstructions seen in the UK. It can be cured in the vast majority of cases by performing an exploratory dacryocystorhinostomy and by carefully separating the adhesions or membrane from around the internal common opening of the common canaliculus. This manoeuvre is facilitated by passing a canalicular probe to tent up the membrane. Great care must be taken not to damage the valves or mucosa surrounding the opening. Once patency has been secured, the canaliculi should be intubated with fine nylon (no. 10 Portex) or silicone (e.g. O'Donoghue) tubes. These are then passed through the rhinostomy and secured together at the external nares, where they are left for at least 3 months. This type of obstruction can usually be identified on the preoperative dacryocystogram, where the common canaliculus fills with dye.

LATERAL OR FIBROUS OBSTRUCTION

In the remaining one-third of cases the common canaliculus is obstructed by pericanalicular fibrosis lateral to the sac. In the UK, the sac is usually normal and the cause of the obstruction is obscure. Worldwide, the usual aetiology is trachoma. The common canaliculus does not fill on the dacryocystogram.

This type of obstruction can usually be permanently relieved by the operation of canaliculodacryocystorhinostomy (CDCR).

CANALICULODACRYOCYSTORHINOSTOMY

(Fig 8.2)

Principle

The junction between patent and obstructed canaliculus is identified in the tissues lateral to the tear sac. The obliterated canaliculus is resected and the patent canaliculus anastomosed to the nose using the sac as a bridge.

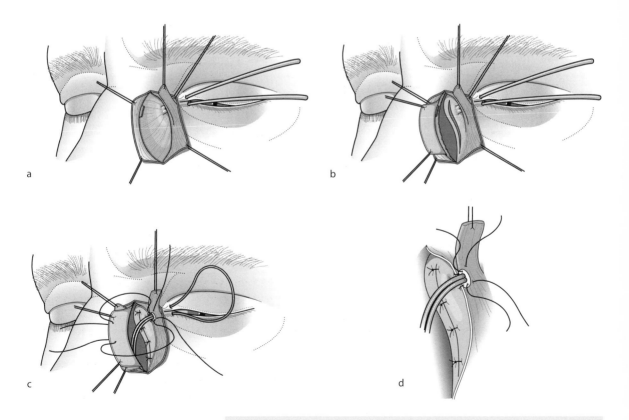

a

b

c

d

Figure 8.2

Indications

Obstruction of the common or individual canaliculi lateral to the sac where there is at least 7 mm of patent canaliculus present.

Method

1. Make a skin incision as for a DCR.
2. Identify the superficial part of the medial palpebral ligament and divide it.
3. Reflect the ligament laterally to expose the anterior surface of the fundus of the sac, being careful not to disturb the periosteum over the anterior lacrimal crest.
4. Place probes in the upper and lower canaliculus.
5. Follow the deep surface of the medial palpebral ligament to identify the common canaliculus as it emerges from the reflected part of that structure (Fig. 8.2a). This is facilitated by gently manipulating the canalicular probes.
6. Clear the superior, inferior and anterior aspects of the common canaliculus from the surrounding tissues. Depending on the amount of patent canaliculus present, the section can be carried laterally into the lid as necessary. It should be pursued until the operator is satisfied that the patent canaliculus is sufficiently mobilised to effect an anastomosis.
7. The periosteum is now divided over the anterior lacrimal crest, the sac reflected laterally, and a large bony rhinostomy created.
8. Incise the tear sac along its anterior aspect close to the junction with the common canaliculus, from the fundus to the naso-lacrimal duct (Fig. 8.2b).
9. Inspect the internal common opening of the common canaliculus to confirm that the obstruction is not of the membranous variety. If it is, proceed as above.
10. If the common canaliculus is obliterated by fibrous tissue, incise the patent common or individual canaliculi and immediately intubate them with fine nylon or silicone tubing.
11. If one canaliculus is absent, the tubing can be passed through the relevant lid using a 19-gauge needle to define a track for it. This must be achieved before attempting to intubate the patent canaliculus.
12. Using the tubing to help with the manipulations, anastomose the posterior margin of the canaliculus to the adjacent sac mucosa with two or three fine long-acting absorbable sutures. The sac may need to be trimmed to give good apposition.
13. Rotate the more medial sac flap posteriorly, and incise the nasal mucosa to create a large anterior and a small posterior flap. The sac is entirely incorporated in the posterior anastomosis.
14. After passing the canalicular tubing through the rhinostomy, anastomose the anterior nasal mucosal flap directly to the anterior aspect of the canaliculus. It is best to position two or three sutures before attempting to secure the knots (Fig. 8.2c).

15. Insert further sutures to join the anterior nasal mucosal flap to the adjacent tissues and reattach the medial palpebral tendon.
16. Close the skin and secure the canalicular tubing at the anterior nares. Leave the tubes in situ for at least 3 months.

Complications

As for DCR. If the tubes start to cut through the canaliculae they should be removed. If the canaliculae block again consider repeating the procedure or lacrimal bypass surgery.

BYPASS SURGERY (Fig 8.3)

Principle

To insert a plastic or glass tube between the inner canthus and nose and thus provide an artificial passageway for the drainage of tears.

Indications

The presence of persistent epiphora in a patient who has no canalicular function. This may be due to congenital absence, physical or irradiational injury, or infections such as herpes simplex or trachoma which obliterate the canaliculi. Adverse drug reactions are sometimes responsible, such as occur in the Stevens–Johnson syndrome. Occasionally, it may be justifiable to insert a bypass tube into a patient with an intact canalicular system but in whom the function has been lost, e.g. in a facial palsy.

Method

1. Perform a DCR in the normal manner up to the point when the posterior mucosal flaps have been sutured (stages 1–14).
2. Inspect the internal opening of the common canaliculus and pass a fine probe retrogradely up it to ensure that there is no

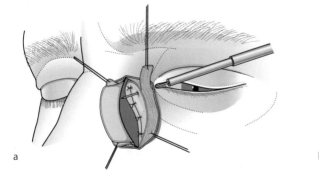
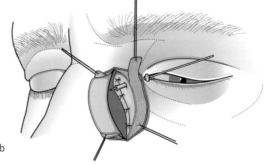

a
b

Figure 8.3

possibility of performing a retrograde canaliculostomy, which may be preferable to the insertion of a bypass tube.

3. Inspect the inner canthus to decide where the lateral end of the tube is to be positioned. There are two possibilities. If the punctum and ampulla are intact the tube can be positioned so that it lies in the posterior lamella of the lid, having carried out a three-snip procedure on the lower punctum. Alternatively, partially or totally excise the caruncle, taking care not to damage the adjacent conjunctiva, and position the tube in the caruncular bed.

4. Define the tract of the tube by pushing a needle such as a Kirschner wire from the inner canthus to the sac in the region of the internal common opening. The direction should be slightly downwards and such that it avoids the anterior end of the middle turbinate.

5. Enlarge the tract to accommodate the tube either by slipping a Graefe knife along the side of the needle or, more conveniently, by passing a 2.25 mm trephine over the needle and removing a core of tissue from around it.

6. Slip a 240 polyethylene tube with an expanded lateral end into position over the needle and trim its medial end so that it lies just short of the nasal septum (Fig. 8.3).

7. Secure the lateral end of the tube to the lid margin with a suture and close the DCR in the normal manner (stages 15–18, p 171).

8. About a week later, remove the plastic tube and replace it with a 2 mm glass tube some 12–16 mm in length. The lateral end of the tube should have a cuff of about 3–4 mm in diameter and its medial end should be expanded to 2.25 mm.

Complications

As for DCR. If the bypass tube is dislodged or lost it must be replaced as immediately as possible or the tract will close. If the tract cannot be dilated and the tube reinserted it will need to be replaced surgically by repeating stages 4–8. If the tube becomes buried in the wound and the epiphora recurs, it can be removed when and if the procedure is repeated.

The by-pass tube can cause granuloma formation. These are usually controlled by excision with cautery to the vascular pedicle and cleaning the tube.

Facial palsy and corneal exposure

9

Acute facial nerve or Bell's palsy is usually idiopathic but some cases are associated with herpes and other viral infections. Facial palsy can also occur as a result of trauma including surgical trauma, tumours such as acoustic neuromas and from a variety of conditions affecting the 7th nerve anywhere along its intra- or extracranial course. Patients should be examined and if necessary investigated to try and establish the cause of the palsy. If it is thought to be idiopathic Bell's palsy they should probably be treated empirically with systemic antiviral therapy and possibly systemic steroids.

ACUTE CORNEAL EXPOSURE

The medical treatment of corneal exposure involves using lubricants such as drops, gels or ointment as frequently as necessary to control symptoms and signs. At night the eyelids can be taped together and padded closed. Various moist chambers can be tried, the simplest of which is to tape cling film around the orbital rim.

Complications

There is always the risk of a corneal abrasion if the eyelids have been closed with a pad or tape etc.

BOTULINUM TOXIN TO LEVATOR MUSCLE

Principle

The levator muscle is paralysed with an injection of botulinum toxin which induces a ptosis. This protects the cornea for up to 3 months.

Indications

Acute corneal exposure which is not adequately controlled by lubricants and is likely to recover spontaneously. It can only be used if the patient can see adequately with the other eye and is likely to be able to manage for some time with uniocular vision.

Method

1. Apply local anaesthetic drops to the conjunctival sac.
2. Evert the lid and give the botulinum toxin above the upper border of the tarsus into the subaponeurotic space just lateral to the midline. If Dysport is used give about 30 units.
3. Continue with medical treatment until the ptosis occurs which may take about 3 days.

Complications

Vertical diplopia can occur from the botulinum toxin diffusing to affect the superior rectus muscle. Very rarely this may lead to a long-standing vertical diplopia but it usually recovers spontaneously.

TEMPORARY TARSORRHAPHY (Figs 9.1, 9.2)

Principle

The two eyelids are sutured together with the excision of little or no eyelid tissue so that when the tarsorrhaphy is undone the lid margins are relatively normal.

Indications

Temporary corneal protection which leaves the visual axis clear. The type of tarsorrhaphy depends on where the maximum protection is required. An extensive lateral tarsorrhaphy can cause a significant loss of the lateral field of vision. The 'central' or 'pillar' tarsorrhaphy avoids this if performed just lateral to the lacrimal puncta (see Fig 9.2f). In this position it also supports the lower lid and helps to correct a paralytic ectropion. It can be performed anywhere along the lid margin to give corneal protection where it is most required, but obviously it will affect vision most if it involves the centre of the lid.

LATERAL TARSORRHAPHY (Fig 9.1)

Method

1. Mark the length of tarsorrhaphy required on the upper and lower lids.
2. Hold each lid with skin hooks at the lateral canthus and just medial to the proposed medial end of the tarsorrhaphy.
3. Make a very shallow incision through the grey line.
4. Excise enough conjunctiva from the lid margin posterior to the grey-line incision to leave a raw surface (Fig. 9.1a).
5. Suture the raw surfaces of the two lids together with mattress sutures tied over bolsters on the skin of the upper and lower lids (Fig. 9.1b).
6. Leave these sutures for 2–3 weeks.
   Note: a) If there is any difficulty in holding the lids together, make a conjunctival incision at the upper border of the upper

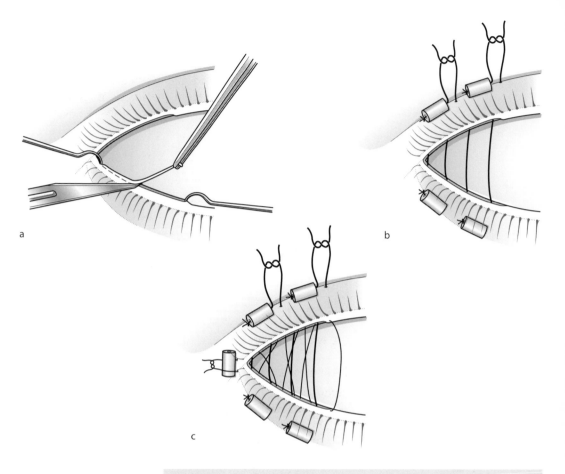

Figure 9.1

tarsus and lower border of the lower and free the lid retractors. Be careful in the upper lid not to damage the lacrimal gland or its ductules. b) If a temporary lateral tarsorrhaphy has pulled apart prematurely and needs to be redone, ensure adequate freeing of the lid retractors and suture the raw surfaces of the lids together with a continuous nylon pull-out suture in addition to the mattress sutres (Fig. 9.1c).

Complications

Limitation of temporal visual field. Risk of trichiasis when the tarsorrhaphy is reversed.

CENTRAL/PILLAR TARSORRHAPHY (Fig 9.2)

Method –

1. Make an incision the length of the required tarsorrhaphy through the grey-line of both eyelids using a no. 11 blade (Fig 9.2a).

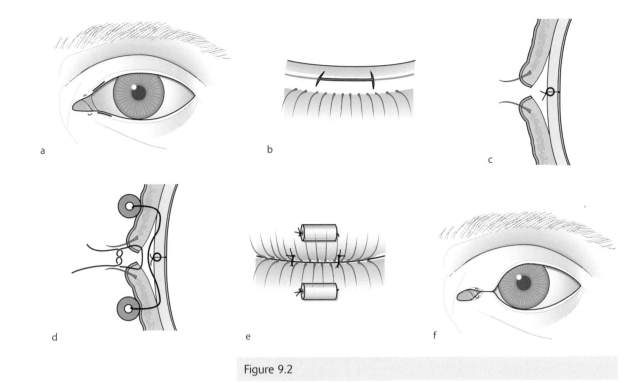

Figure 9.2

2. At each end of this incision make a very small cut at right angles to the lid margin but not through its extremities. This makes the wound H-shaped (Fig. 9.2b).
3. Evert each split lid margin and suture the raw surfaces of the two tarsal plates together with a buried 6 '0' long-acting absorbable suture. This must not extend through the full thickness of the tarsal plates or it may abrade the cornea (Fig. 9.2c).
4. Pass a mattress suture through the centre of the wound and tie it over bolsters on the skin of the upper and lower lids.
5. Suture the everted anterior lamellae together with a skin suture to complete the three-layer closure (Fig. 9.2d,e).
6. Remove the mattress suture at 2–3 weeks (Fig 9.2f).
    Note: both a lateral and a central/pillar tarsorrhaphy can be left as a permanent tarsorrhaphy but the interpalpebral junction will tend to stretch usually more with a pillar tarsorrhaphy than with a lateral tarsorrhaphy.

Complications

There is less risk of trichiasis and eyelid margin distortion when a central/pillar tarsorrhaphy is reversed than when a lateral tarsorrhaphy is reversed because no lid tissue has been excised.

ESTABLISHED CHRONIC 7TH NERVE PALSY

- Corneal protection
- Paralytic ectropion
- Cosmesis

I. CORNEAL PROTECTION

Corneal exposure in 7th nerve palsy is due to poor eyelid closure. This is aggravated by eyelid retraction caused by the unopposed action of the levator muscle. The retraction can be treated with an upper lid retractor recession. Eyelid closure can be improved in various ways including burying a weight in the upper lid. This is particularly valuable if there is a poor Bell's phenomenon and marked lagophthalmos. Corneal exposure will be improved the more the palpebral aperture is reduced. In addition to lowering the upper lid, the lower lid can be raised in various ways and the horizontal palpebral aperture reduced with a combination of a medial canthoplasty and lateral and/or other tarsorrhaphies.

SYSTEM FOR ESTABLISHED CORNEAL EXPOSURE

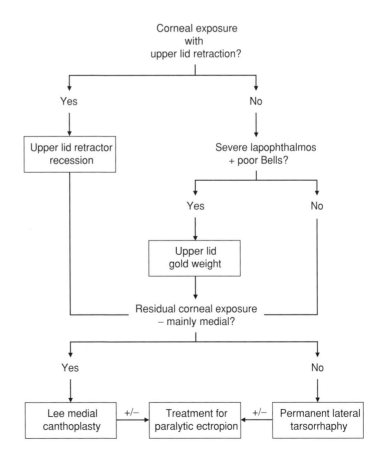

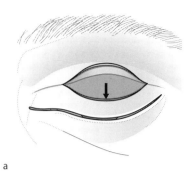

a

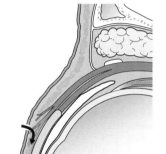

UPPER LID RETRACTOR RECESSION (p 196)

Principle

The upper lid retractors are recessed to counteract their overaction which is caused by the paralysis of their antagonist, the orbicularis muscle.

Indications

Upper lid retraction and corneal exposure from 7th nerve palsy.

Method

- Mild
  - Posterior approach upper lid retractor recession (p 196)
- More severe
  - Blepharotomy. If under local anaesthesia (p 198)
  - Adjustable sutures. If under general anaesthesia (p 107).

Complications

Lid too high, too low, poor contour, asymmetric skin crease.

UPPER LID GOLD WEIGHT (Fig 9.3)

Principle

A gold weight is positioned under the skin and orbicularis muscle on the anterior tarsal surface via a skin crease incision. It assists eyelid closure through gravity. Different weights are temporarily attached to the upper lid with double sided tape to identify which one best achieves adequate eyelid closure while still maintaining a clear pupillary axis in the primary position of gaze.

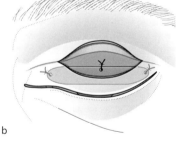

b

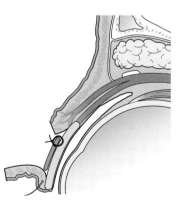

Figure 9.3

Indications

Corneal exposure from 7th nerve palsy etc. without significant lid retraction and with normal sensation.

Method

1. Make a skin crease incision and expose the anterior surface of the tarsus down to the lash roots (Fig 9.3a).
2. Place the predetermined weight on the anterior tarsal surface.
3. Suture the weight to the anterior tarsus with permanent sutures such as 6 '0' nylon passed through holes in the weight (Fig 9.3b).
4. Close the orbicularis muscle with buried 6 '0' long-acting absorbable sutures and close the skin separately making a two layer closure over the weight for extra security.
5. Cover with systemic antibiotics.

Complications

Extrusion, dislocation, bulky lid, visible colour of implant through lid, raised skin crease, reduced vision from irregular corneal astigmatism.

Extrusion may occur as with any foreign body. It is more frequent if there is a sensory defect. The risk of dislocation is reduced if the shape of the weight conforms accurately to the curve of the tarsus and if the weight is sutured to the anterior tarsal surface. Although gold is traditional it may be bulky, its colour visible and its necessary vertical height may cause the skin crease to be a little high. New platinum weights have been developed which being heavier are smaller and possibly a better colour match which may improve these disadvantages. The eyelid weight may distort the cornea causing irregular astigmatism and poor vision.

LEE MEDIAL CANTHOPLASTY (See p 78, Fig 4.17)

Principle

The eyelids are sutured together medial to the lacrimal puncta to improve corneal protection by reducing both the horizontal palpebral aperture and the increased vertical interpalpebral distance at the medial canthus.

Indications

Corneal exposure mainly affecting the medial cornea.

Method

See p 78.

PERMANENT LATERAL TARSORRHAPHY (Fig 9.4)

Principle

The two eyelids are overlapped laterally and sutured together with the excision of tissue to limit the soft tissue distraction that occurs with a temporary tarsorrhaphy. This reduces the horizontal palpebral aperture improving corneal protection and supports the lower lid.

Indications

Chronic corneal exposure e.g. established 7th nerve palsy; lower lid support after retractor lengthening; camouflage of proptosis; chronic corneal and tear film abnormalities.

Method

1. Mark the extent of the planned tarsorrhaphy (Fig 9.4a).

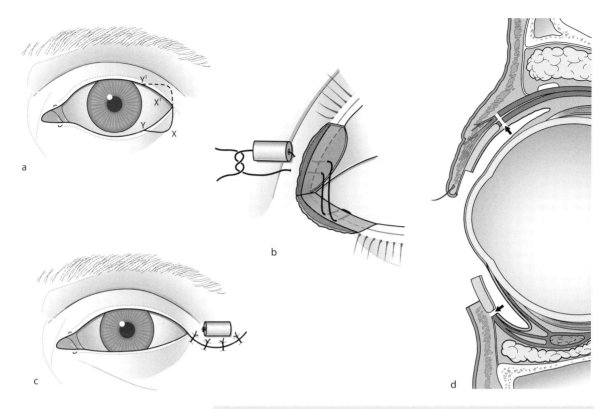

Figure 9.4

2. Split the lower lid at the grey-line and excise a curved half-moon portion of the anterior lamella, i.e. skin and orbicularis, with the lower lid margin, as shown in the diagram (Fig 9.4b).
3. Excise a similar curved half-moon shape of the posterior part of the tarsal plate with the tarsal conjunctiva and with the lid margin epithelium from the upper lid. The best union between the lids is obtained if only partial thickness tarsus is excised.
4. Suture the raw surfaces of the two lids together with a suture tied over a bolster on the skin (Fig 9.4b).
5. Suture the upper lid margin to the cut lower lid skin edge to reinforce the closure. Use interrupted sutures and remove them after about 7 days (Fig 9.4c).
6. Leave the suture tied over the bolster for 2–3 weeks.

   Note: a. If the tarsorrhaphy is under tension, free the upper and lower lid retractors (Fig 9.4d).

   b. This tarsorrhaphy can be done anywhere on the lid or can be extended as a total tarsorrhaphy.

Complications

Limitation of temporal visual field. If a 'permanent' lateral tarsorrhaphy has to be opened there is a significant risk of lid margin distortion and trichiasis.

Cosmesis. This will be very poor and the tarsorrhaphy may not hold if a permanent lateral tarsorrhaphy is used to try and correct corneal exposure without recessing the lid retractors when there is lid retraction and proptosis.

II. PARALYTIC ECTROPION

The paralysed lower lid requires support for the paralysis and tightening to correct the laxity. This may be easily achieved with a Lee medial canthoplasty and lateral canthal suture or may require the addition of other procedures. The choice of which operations are necessary in any individual depends both on the physical examination and the symptoms. If the patient is complaining of epiphora from the lateral canthus quite clearly he needs to have lateral canthal surgery.

The system, management scheme and operative headings are repeated here from p 77 for ease of reference.

SYSTEM FOR PARALYTIC LOWER LID ECTROPION

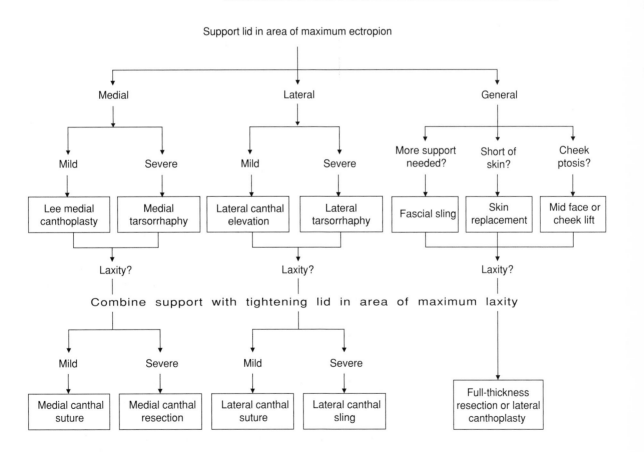

MANAGEMENT

1. Support
   a. Medial:
      - Lee medial canthoplasty
      - medial tarsorrhaphy
   b. Lateral:
      - lateral canthal elevation
      - lateral tarsorrhaphy
   c. General:
      - fascial sling
2. Tighten
   a. Medial:
      - medial canthal suture
      - medial canthal resection
   b. Lateral:
      - lateral canthal suture
      - lateral tarsal strip
3. Correction of secondary changes to support lid:
      - skin graft
      - cheek/mid face lift.

LEE MEDIAL CANTHOPLASTY (p 78, Fig 4.17)

Principle

The eyelids are sutured together medial to the lacrimal puncta to support the lower lid and reduce the increased vertical interpalpebral distance at the medial canthus and to bring the lacrimal puncta into the tear film.

LATERAL CANTHAL ELEVATION (p 80, Fig 4.19)

Principle

The lateral canthal tendon is freed from the lateral orbital wall and the orbital septum. Any structures tethering it are released. It is reattached to the periosteum of the lateral orbital wall at a higher level to support the lower lid.

FASCIAL SLING (p 219, Fig 11.10)

Principle

A strip of fascia is passed through the lid from the medial canthal tendon to the lateral orbital wall.

SKIN GRAFT (p 74)

Principle

If the 7th nerve palsy is long-standing, secondary changes of skin contraction can occur which increase the paralytic ectropion and lid retraction. These may require skin grafting, often with a lateral canthoplasty to further support and to tighten the lid. A full thickness lid resection can also be used to tighten the lid.

CHEEK PTOSIS

Principle

In cases of long-standing 7th nerve palsy the weight of the paralysed cheek leads to a cheek ptosis. This may require correction with a cheek or mid face lift. See p 248.

TIGHTEN LID

Principle

A paralysed lower lid requires support for the paralysis and tightening to correct the laxity. The horizontal lid tightening procedures have been covered in Chapter 4 and can be combined with any of the lid supporting procedures described here.

III. COSMESIS

Patient with 7th nerve palsy are often very distressed about their appearance. This can often be significantly improved by raising the brow, lowering the upper lid and improving the paralytic ectropion.

- Direct brow lift, p 245
- The correction of lid retraction, p 196
- Correction of paralytic lower lid ectropion, p 76.

EPIPHORA IN 7TH NERVE PALSY

AETIOLOGY

Epiphora is usually due to a combination of reflex tearing from corneal exposure and failure of lacrimal drainage due to a paralytic lower lid ectropion and failure of the blink and lacrimal pump mechanism. It can be aggravated by aberrant 7th nerve regeneration.

MANAGEMENT

Treat the corneal exposure; correct the paralytic ectropion; improve tear drainage; consider botulinum toxin for aberrant 7th nerve regeneration.

The tear drainage can be improved with (1) dacryocystorhinostomy and (2) a lacrimal bypass (Jones) tube.

TREATMENT

The treatment of epiphora in 7th nerve palsy is first to reduce the reflex production of excess tears as much as possible by treating any corneal exposure, lid retraction and lagophthalmos. Any lower lid malposition and ectropion should then be corrected and the effect of gravity on tear drainage improved by raising the lateral part of the lid. The lacrimal puncta must be inverted into the tear lake. The lacrimal drainage itself can then be improved by carrying out a dacryocystorhinostomy to reduce any resistance to tear drainage. If this does not relieve the epiphora sufficiently a lacrimal bypass (Jones) tube can be considered.

CORNEAL EXPOSURE

Corneal exposure may occur from many causes other than 7th nerve palsy e.g. trauma (p 161), eyelid tissue defects (Chapter 6), thyroid eye disease, proptosis, lid retraction, restricted ocular movements, tear film and corneal abnormalities. Lubricants, contact lenses, moist chambers, etc. may help at least in the short term and surgery should be aimed at improving lid closure over the globe as described elsewhere in this book. If the area of corneal exposure does not involve the pupillary axis and the lids cannot be made to cover the relevant area of exposure satisfactorily, it may be reasonable to consider a conjunctival flap.

CONJUNCTIVAL FLAP

Principle

A flap of vascularised conjunctiva is used to cover part of the cornea.

Indications

Corneal exposure that cannot be corrected with lid surgery; indolent corneal ulcer, etc.

Method

1. Scrape the epithelium off the exposed cornea to provide a raw base for the conjunctiva.

2. Raise a suitable flap of conjunctiva, usually a direct advancement from the limbus or a bipedicle flap, and suture it directly over the defect with 7 '0' long-acting absorbable sutures.

Complications

There is a marked tendency for the flap to retract and it must be very extensively undermined to try and prevent this. This can lead to shortening of the conjunctival fornices.

Thyroid eye disease

10

Thyrotoxicosis is an incompletely understood condition in which the autoregulatory control of the thyroid breaks down. An autoimmune reaction occurs which leads to excessive stimulation of the thyroid, excess thyroxine production, increased fibroblast activity and the laying down of mucopolysaccharides and aminoglycans. This may affect various parts of the body, especially the orbit. The inter-relationship between thyrotoxicosis, its treatment and the onset and severity of any orbitopathy is not understood but various factors are known to increase the risk of orbitopathy such as smoking in females.

It has been clearly recognised for many years that there is an active inflammatory phase of thyroid eye disease characterised by combinations of symptoms and signs of acute inflammation Classically the signs of acute inflammation are heat, pain, redness, swelling and loss of function. In acute thyroid orbitopathy this translates into ocular irritation, discomfort and possibly pain, conjunctival redness, vascular engorgement and swelling, ocular motility disturbance, corneal signs, lid retraction, proptosis and visual impairment. Various combinations of these symptoms and signs form the basis of different classifications of the severity of the ophthalmopathy. The active phase lasts on average 18 months but this is very variable. It is succeeded by the static or quiescent phase in which the condition is stable.

Treatment in the active phase aims to control (1) the thyrotoxicosis (2) the ophthalmopathy and (3) the complications. It is hoped that such control may reduce the length of the active phase and induce quiescence which can then be managed according to a staged protocol. This involves assessing and if necessary carrying out surgery in the following order: (1) orbital decompression, (2) squint surgery, (3) eyelid surgery.

SYSTEM FOR THYROID EYE DISEASE

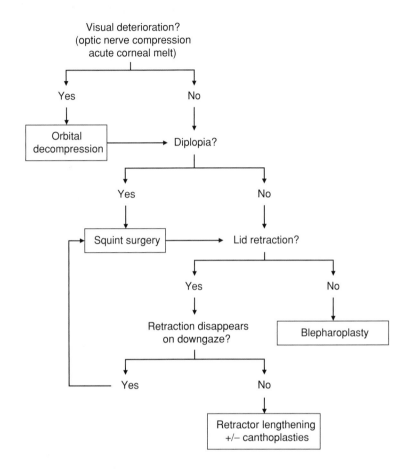

MANAGEMENT

- Active phase
  1. Thyrotoxicosis
  2. Ophthalmopathy
  3. Complications
- Static quiescent phase
  1. Orbital decompression
  2. Squint surgery
  3. Lid surgery.

THYROTOXICOSIS

The management of thyrotoxicosis involves suppression, blocking or ablating the thyroid. This can be achieved by various combinations of drugs, radioactive iodine and/or surgery with thyroxine replacement.

ACTIVE OPHTHALMOPATHY

Control of the active ophthalmopathy involves systemic steroids with retro-orbital irradiation and possibly immunosuppression. The aim of treatment in the acute phase is to make the patient comfortable, try to prevent complications and to limit the duration and extent of the active phase. Although systemic steroids, retro-orbital irradiation and immunosuppression can have a dramatic effect on reducing the signs of active inflammation, it is not yet clear whether this has any effect on permanently switching off the active phase of the condition and achieving the static quiescent phase any quicker than would have happened spontaneously.

If the condition is mild and all that is needed is to keep the patient comfortable with lubricants, it may be reasonable not to give any systemic treatment. If the condition is more active retro-orbital irradiation is effective but should be avoided in diabetics. The irradiation takes some time to act and it is usual to start a patient who requires treatment on systemic steroids and to give the retro-orbital irradiation at the same time. Systemic steroids are quick acting and very effective at reducing the acute inflammatory reaction. It is preferable to limit their long-term use because of their side effects. Immunosuppression may allow the dose of systemic steroids to be reduced. This may be particularly valuable with diabetics whose condition may be unstabilised by systemic steroids. If complications occur during the active phase of the ophthalmopathy they are treated as detailed below with a combination of aggressive medical therapy and if necessary orbital decompression and upper lid lowering.

CONTROL OF ACTIVE OPHTHALMOPATHY COMPLICATIONS

The main complications in the active phase of the condition are corneal exposure and optic nerve compression. Minor symptoms can be controlled with lubricant drops and ointment. Systemic steroids may control more severe symptoms both of corneal exposure and optic nerve compression but some patients will require a surgical orbital decompression – sometimes as a relatively acute emergency. The state of the cornea may need to be monitored closely as an acute corneal melt can occur depending on the degree of lid retraction and proptosis. Optic nerve compression can be monitored by assessing colour vision, visual acuity and in severe cases by pupillary signs. MRI and CT scans will demonstrate the degree of congestion at the orbital apex. If corneal exposure is sufficiently severe it is justifiable to lower the upper lid with an upper lid retractor recession in the acute phase provided it is accepted that the lid level may need to be adjusted subsequently in the quiescent phase.

ORBITAL DECOMPRESSION

Principle

The orbit can be decompressed medically with high doses of systemic steroids and surgically either by removing orbital bones or reducing the orbital fat. There are various surgical approaches for bony orbital wall decompression including the coronal, transantral, caruncular, lateral canthal and subciliary blepharoplasty approach. The lateral canthal and subciliary blepharoplasty approach will allow access to the orbital floor, medial and lateral orbital walls and is described on p 214.

Orbital decompression by removing orbital fat can be achieved by exploring mainly the superomedial and inferolateral quadrants of the orbit. Although orbits can be decompressed in this way it is not easy to assess the extent of fat removal necessary to achieve a given degree of reduction of the proptosis.

Indications

An acute orbital wall decompression may be required if systemic steroids have either failed to control or are contraindicated in the management of optic nerve compression or acute corneal melt. More often the indication for surgical orbital decompression is 'significant proptosis' which can be a cosmetic as well as functional defect. The extent of the proptosis for which a decompression is required can be variably defined but may be 25 mm or less. Orbital fat decompression may be of value if the orbital muscles can be shown on MRI or CT scan to be relatively normal in size. Orbital bone decompression is certainly indicated if the muscles are enlarged, which they usually are. Some surgeons combine orbital bone and orbital fat decompression.

Method

Steps 1–4 as for lateral canthal approach to orbital floor/swinging eyelid flap (p 214, see Fig 11.7).

5. Elevate the periosteum superiorly over the orbital rim and continue the elevation along the orbital floor extending up the medial wall. Support the periosteum and orbital contents with a malleable orbital retractor.
6. Fracture the thin orbital floor bone with heavy artery forceps and deroof the infraorbital nerve.
7. Remove as much of the orbital floor and medial wall bone as required but leave the strut of bone anteriorly at the junction of the orbital floor and medial wall posterior to the lacrimal sac. This helps to prevent hypoglobus.
8. Release the orbital fat by making a series of longitudinal incisions through the orbital periosteum starting posteriorly and

coming forward. These incision must be kept shallow and not carried too far anteriorly to avoid damage to the infraorbital structures and inferior suspensory ligament of the globe.

9. Close the periosteum with 4 '0' long-acting absorbable sutures.
10. Follow lateral canthal approach to orbital floor stages 8–10 (p 216).

Complications

Loss of sight; squint; anaesthesia or change in sensation in the distribution of the infraorbital nerve; over- and undercorrection. With any orbital procedure the vision and pupillary reactions must be monitored postoperatively. If the vision is deteriorating and the pupil enlarging the wound must be explored.

SQUINT SURGERY

Extraocular muscle imbalance should be monitored during the acute phase of thyroid eye disease. If diplopia is uncontrollable the patient may need to occlude one eye. When the orbitopathy is stable and any orbital decompression surgery has been carried out if appropriate, diplopia should be corrected with squint surgery. Orthoptic assessment and Hess charts etc. should first demonstrate that the ocular position has remained stable for at least 3 and preferably 6 or even 9 months. The usual cause of diplopia is infiltration and scarring of the extraocular muscles. Any muscle may be infiltrated, thickened, fibrosed and tight but the inferior rectus is most commonly involved. This may cause secondary upper lid retraction which becomes more marked when the patient looks up and disappears on down gaze. This is in contradistinction to lid retraction caused by proptosis and infiltration scarring and thickening of the upper lid retractors in which the lid retraction is constant or even increased on downgaze.

The inferior rectus muscle is particularly suitable for a recession with adjustable sutures, but any recession of this muscle tends to cause or aggravate lower lid retraction. This can be reduced at surgery by freeing the lower lid retractors from the inferior rectus as completely as possible and by putting the lower lid on traction for 24–48 hours postoperatively. Established lower lid retraction may require management with a spacer as described below.

EYELID SURGERY

   I. Upper lid retractor lengthening
  II. Lower lid retractor lengthening
 III. Canthoplasty
 IV. Blepharoplasty

I. UPPER LID RETRACTOR LENGTHENING

Principle

The upper lid is lowered by recessing the upper lid retractors. The lid will only drop is there is sufficient skin and conjunctiva and the lid retraction is not secondary to inferior rectus muscle restriction (see under Squint Surgery above).

Indications

The correction of lid retraction which may be required for corneal exposure or cosmetic reasons. Lid retraction may be caused by thyroid problems, 7th nerve palsy, proptosis from any cause, trauma or be consecutive following excessive ptosis correction etc. If the lid is lowered via a posterior approach this will create a jatrogenic 'levator disinsertion' and the skin crease will rise. This does not matter in mild or bilateral cases but may be significant in more severe unilateral cases when an anterior approach blepharotomy is preferable. If the patient requires general anaesthesia, it is difficult to assess how much to recess the retractors and adjustable sutures are valuable as they give some postoperative control of lid level and contour. It is rarely necessary to consider other methods of lowering an upper eyelid such as a Z myotomy or the addition of a spacer. The addition of a spacer can however be useful in cases of recurrent lid retraction which have proved resistant to control by other methods.

- Mild retraction
  - Posterior approach retractor recession
- More severe retraction.
  - Local anaesthesia: blepharotomy.
  - General anaesthesia: adjustable sutures.
- Recurrent retraction.
  - Anterior approach retractor recession with spacer.

POSTERIOR APPROACH UPPER LID RETRACTOR RECESSION (Fig 10.1)

Method

1. Insert a traction suture through tubing. Evert the lid over a Desmarres' retractor and make an incision just above the tarsus (Fig 10.1a,b).
2. Deepen the incision until the lid is lowered to a level that is as much below as it was previously above the final level that it is hoped to be achieved.
   Note: the lid lowering effect is increased if the anterior surface of the tarsus is cleaned. It is often necessary to cut the lateral horn of the levator, particularly in thyroid patients.

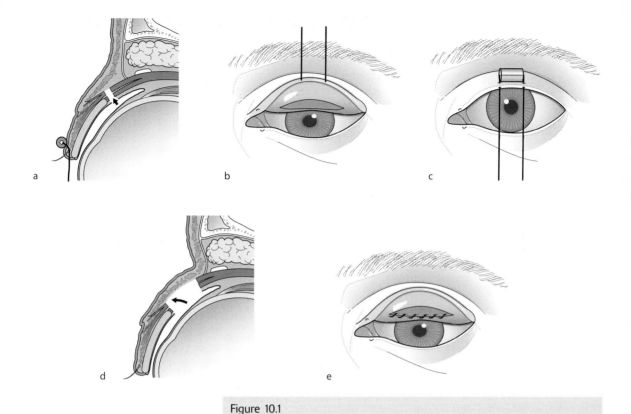

Figure 10.1

3. Tape the traction suture to the cheek to pull the upper lid down (Fig 10.1c).
4. Remove the traction suture after 24 hours.
5. When the lid achieves the desired height, maintain it there by massage and lid traction. This may be required for up to 3–4 months before the lid level stabilises.

Note: The effectiveness of the upper lid retractor recession can be increased by suturing the conjunctiva and retractors to the overlying preseptal orbicularis muscle with a continuous fine long-acting absorbable suture or a pull-out 6 '0' nylon suture which can be removed after a few days (Fig 10.1d,e).

Complications

Eyelid level too high, too low, poor contour, raised skin crease, post-operative bleeding from the open conjunctival wound. This usually stops with pressure but it is wise to warn the patient of the possibility of bleeding.

BLEPHAROTOMY (Fig 10.2)

Method

1. Make a skin crease incision and deepen it through skin and orbicularis muscle down to the anterior surface of the tarsal plate (Fig 10.2a).
2. Check the lid level. Then start cutting through all the remaining tissues immediately above the upper border of the tarsal plate, i.e. aponeurosis, Muller's muscle and conjunctiva. In thyroid patients start this incision in the lateral third of the lid. In other patients start where the lid retraction is most marked (Fig 10.2b).
3. Extend this full thickness incision medially and laterally until the lid level is the same as the other side or at the desired level. Leave a small bridge of conjunctiva at the point of maximum eyelid curvature, which is usually the junction of the medial third with the lateral two-thirds of the lid (Fig 10.2c). Keep checking the lid height. If the level drops too low, suture the conjunctiva back together with a 6 '0' long-acting absorbable suture placed where it is desired to have more elevation. If the lid level will not drop sufficiently despite cutting the conjunctiva com-

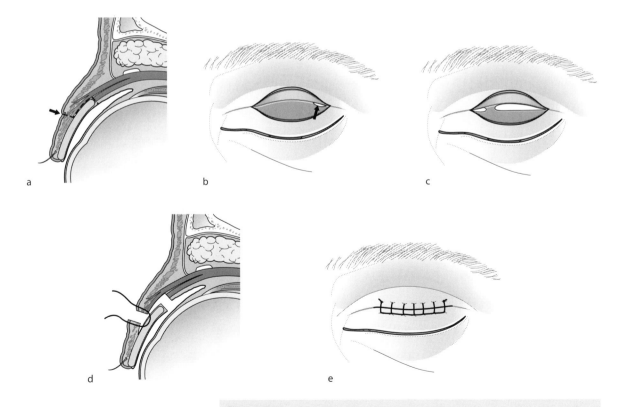

a   b   c

d   e

Figure 10.2

pletely free the levator muscle and cut its medial and lateral horns.

4. When satisfied with the lid level and contour, close the skin and orbicularis muscle and pick up a bite of the anterior tarsal surface with a running locked 5 '0' long-acting absorbable suture or black silk suture. (Fig 10.1d) This suture needs to be carefully positioned to prevent fistula formation. (Fig 10.1e)

   Note: If the skin crease appears to be too high, open the orbital septum and free the preaponeurotic fat so that it comes down to the skin crease reforming sutures.

5. Remove the sutures after 10 days. If postoperatively the lid is too high start eyelid traction and massage early and maintain it for three to four months if necessary.

Complications

Eyelid level too high, too low, poor contour, asymmetric skin crease, fistula. If this occurs excise it and carefully resuture the wound.

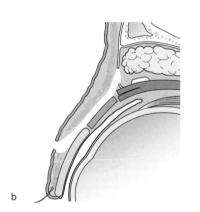
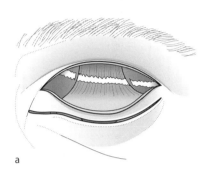

a

ADJUSTABLE SUTURES FOR LID RETRACTION
(See Fig 5.9, p 107)

Method

This is exactly the same technique whether used for the correction of ptosis or lid retraction and is described on p 107.

Complications

Eyelid too high, too low, poor contour, asymmetric skin crease, inflammation and infection of the adjustable sutures. If this occurs the sutures should be removed early and the patient given systemic antibiotics.

b

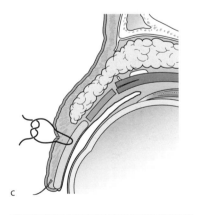

c

ANTERIOR APPROACH UPPER LID RETRACTOR RECESSION WITH SPACER (Fig 10.3)

Method

Stages 1–8 as for anterior approach ptosis surgery (p 100).

9. Cut Whitnall's superior suspensory ligament of the globe (Fig 10.3a).

10. Cut a spacer graft e.g. ear cartilage, sclera etc about 15 mm wide. The height should be about twice the amount of the lid retraction medially and three times the amount laterally.

11. Suture the aponeurosis and Müller's muscle to the edge of the graft with a 6 '0' absorbable suture.

12. Suture the other edge of the graft to the upper border of the tarsus (Fig 10.3b).

13. Free the aponeurotic fat.

Figure 10.3

14. Reform the skin crease with 6 '0' absorbable sutures which pick up the underlying tarsus or graft depending on the height of the skin crease (Fig 10.3c).
15. Put the lid on traction.

Complications

Eyelid level too high, too low, poor contour, asymmetric skin crease, eyelid thickening. The graft can give some thickening of the upper lid which may require later exploration and thinning of the graft. This may occur particularly with ear cartilage grafts, especially if the perichondrium has not been removed sufficiently.

II. LOWER LID RETRACTOR LENGTHENING
(Fig 10.4)

Principle

A graft or 'spacer' is interposed between the cut lid retractors and the lower border of the tarsus. The lid margin cannot be raised beyond the level of the medial and lateral canthal tendons and will only reach this level if there is no excess horizontal lid laxity, some orbicularis

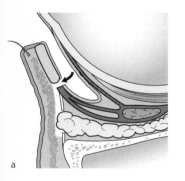
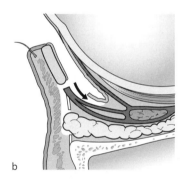
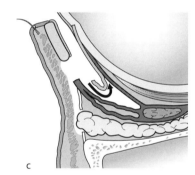

a   b   c

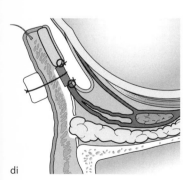
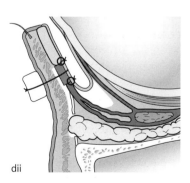
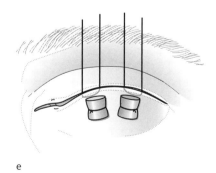

di   dii   e

Figure 10.4

muscle function, and no shortage of lower lid skin. If the globe is proptosed, the lid may require support medially with a canthoplasty and laterally with a tarsorrhaphy or lateral canthal suture. The lid can be raised a little by recessing the retractors without a spacer but the elevation achieved is much greater if a 'spacer' is used. This is possibly because the 'spacer' helps to support the lid as well as keeping the retractors recessed.

Indications

Lid retraction, e.g. dysthyroid; proptosis; trauma; after inferior rectus recession; partial seventh nerve palsy; entropion, if caused by lower lid retractor fibrosis and posterior lamella shortening such as occasionally occurs in dysthyroid patients. The grafts or 'spacers' may be:
- Autogenous
  - e.g. mucous membrane, hard palate, ear cartilage.
- Nonautogenous.
  - Integrateable e.g. Medpor.
  - Nonintegrateable e.g. sclera, Alloderm etc.

Autogenous grafts contract less but have to be harvested.

Method

1. Put two traction sutures through the lid margin.
2. Evert the lid over a Desmarres' retractor.
3. Make an incision through the conjunctiva at the lower border of the tarsus.
4. If the proposed graft has its own mucosal lining (e.g. mucous membrane, hard palate) or will conjunctivalise (e.g. ear cartilage, sclera, Alloderm) cut the lower lid retractors from the tarsus and free them from the preseptal orbicularis muscle in one layer with the conjunctiva. Free the lower lid preaponeurotic fat to be sure that the lower lid retractors are completely disconnected. (Fig 10.4a) The lower lid should no longer move on downgaze if the operation is carried out under local anaesthetic.
5. Cut the graft large enough to fully correct the lid retraction but not so large that it makes the lower lid bulky. A graft of about 2 mm for each mm of lid retraction below the limbus is usually required.
6. Suture the graft to the cut lower lid retractors and conjunctiva below and to the lower border of the tarsus above.
   Note: If the graft does not have a mucosal surface (e.g. ear cartilage, sclera, Alloderm) it can be sutured between the tarsus and the lower lid retractors and covered in conjunctiva. This is more comfortable for the patient and raises the lid more effectively than if the material is left bare. The conjunctiva must first be undermined from the lower lid retractors (Fig 10.4b) and from the inferior suspensory ligament of the fornix to allow it to be mobilised to cover the graft (Fig 10.4c). If the graft is integrateable and relatively stiff such as Medpor it is better inserted via an anterior skin

muscle approach blepharoplasty incision to minimise the risks of exposure and granuloma formation.

7. Pass two double-armed nonabsorbable sutures through the graft, orbicularis and skin (Fig 10.4di) with the conjunctiva if it has been mobilised (Fig 10.4dii). Tie them over bolsters to hold the graft in contact with its bed and to help splint the lid (Fig 10.4d).

   Note: It is often useful to combine lower lid retractor lengthening with a lateral canthal suture or other supporting and elevating procedure.

8. Pull up the lower lid with the traction sutures inserted at the beginning of the operation and tape them to the brow (Fig 10.4e).

9. Remove the traction sutures after 48 hours and the sutures tied over bolsters after 5–7 days.

Complications

Lower lid not high enough, too high (rare), bulky, erosion of foreign material through conjunctiva, granuloma formation.

If the eyelid is not high enough it may be necessary to support the medial and lateral ends of the eyelid with a medial and lateral canthoplasty. The eyelid is rarely too high but if it is or the lid becomes bulky, the graft can be reduced. If foreign material extrudes through the conjunctiva or leads to granuloma formation it should be removed.

III. CANTHOPLASTIES

The horizontal palpebral aperture may be reduced by medial canthoplasty (p 78) and/or lateral tarsorrhaphies (p 178) – these are indicated in thyroid patients with proptosis after a lid retractor lengthening to help raise the lower lid, camouflage the proptosis and improve the tear film. A temporary tarsorrhaphy (p 178) may be helpful in controlling acute corneal exposure, but permanent tarsorrhaphies are not indicated primarily for corneal protection. This is better achieved with lubricants, lid retractor lengthening or orbital decompression.

IV. BLEPHAROPLASTIES

Upper and lower lid blepharoplasties may be performed as described in Chapter 12. The cosmetic benefit in thyroid patients may be less than anticipated because of proptosis and the need to leave enough skin so that the eyelid closure is not limited in patients with a defective tear film. Care must be taken not to remove too much preaponeurotic fat in an attempt to reduce the bulky appearance. This will cause a high skin crease which will be enhanced if the lid is also lowered. The brow fat pad can be reduced but if the patient really wants the bulky appearance improved consideration should be give to an orbital decompression.

Enucleation, evisceration and socket surgery

11

Removal of an eye can have a devastating emotional, psychological and social impact as well as the obvious effect on vision. The physical stigmata of losing an eye can be reduced if an implant is inserted at the time of the enucleation or evisceration. Most socket problems are either related to a volume deficit following enucleation or to a deficit of lining and a contracted socket.

ENUCLEATION WITHOUT IMPLANT (Fig 11.1)

Principle

The complete excision of the eye.

Indications

Blind painful eye; intraocular tumour; trauma; risk of sympathetic ophthalmitis. Although cosmetically the best result is usually achieved if an orbital implant is inserted at the time of the enucleation, there may be occasions e.g. in a very sick patient after trauma, when the quickest simplest complete excision of the eye is indicated.

Method

1. Make a 360° limbal incision through the conjunctiva and Tenon's capsule (Fig 11.1a).
2. Isolate the rectus muscles and tie each muscle with a double-armed 4 '0' long-acting absorbable suture.
3. Cut them from the globe with a cautery or scissors (Fig 11.1b).
4. Cut the superior and inferior oblique muscles.
5. Cut the optic nerve with a wire snare or scissors and complete the enucleation (Fig 11.1c). Proceed with an implant provided that there is no contraindication, e.g. visible extraocular tumour extension, orbital cellulitis, etc.

   Note: use of cautery to cut the muscles and a wire snare for the optic nerve reduces trauma, which is essential when enucleating an eye with a tumour, e.g. a malignant melanoma. It is preferable in these cases not to use a traction suture for the globe as shown in Fig 11.1b, but this suture is very

a

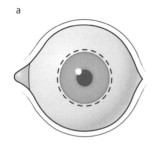

b

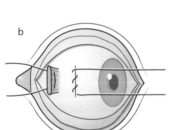

c

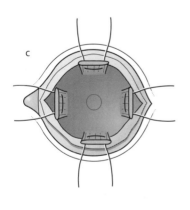

Figure 11.1

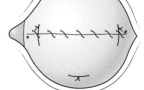

Figure 11.1   cont'd

useful in other circumstances, e.g. when enucleating a soft eye after trauma.

6. If no implant is to be inserted pass the long-acting absorbable sutures from the rectus muscles through Tenon's capsule and the conjunctiva in the superior, medial, inferior and lateral fornices and tie them before closing the conjunctiva (Fig 11.1d). This will improve motility of the fornices and artificial eye. The movement will be further enhanced and the volume deficit improved if an implant is inserted. A conformer or shell should be retained in the socket to maintain the fornices.

Complications

Postenucleation socket syndrome is caused when no implant or an implant with an inadequate volume is inserted at the time of the enucleation.

EVISCERATION WITHOUT IMPLANT (Fig 11.2)

Principle

The ocular contents are removed, leaving the scleral envelope.

Indications

Blind painful eye, panophthalmitis. This is the quickest simplest way of effectively removing an eye provided it does not have an intraocular tumour. If the optic nerve is cut, as with an enucleation, the meninges are opened and there is a theoretical risk of inducing meningitis in patients with panophthalmitis. This was a more serious concern before the antibiotic era.

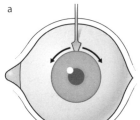

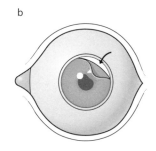

Method

1. Make a stab incision at the limbus with a blade (Fig 11.2a).
2. Excise the cornea with a pair of curved scissors, leaving the conjunctival attachment to the limbus intact to limit the risk of spreading infection by opening tissue planes.
3. Eviscerate the ocular contents with a curved instrument or 'evisceration spoon' (Fig 11.2b).
4. Leave the scleral wound open to drain or close it with a locked running 6 '0' absorbable suture (Fig 11.2c). It will granulate and fibrose to form a firm knot of scleral tissue. The discharge can be reduced with antibiotic drops if necessary.

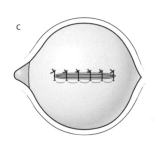

Figure 11.2

Complications

Sympathetic ophthalmitis. An evisceration leaves the sclera and usually some uveal remnants intact. The potential for causing sympathetic ophthalmitis is not totally avoided by removing an eye with an evisceration.

Volume deficit. This will occur if no implant is inserted after an evisceration producing a form of the postenucleation socket syndrome.

ORBITAL IMPLANTS

AUTOGENOUS

– e.g. dermis fat graft.

NONAUTOGENOUS

– Integrateable
– Nonintegrateable

Spherical implant shapes are preferred because they have the greatest volume for a given surface area but transfer of movement to the artificial eye may be less than with other implant shapes.

The commonest autogenous implant is a dermis fat graft. This has the advantage that it will not extrude, which is particularly valuable after trauma. It has the disadvantage that the graft will absorb to an unknown and variable extent, possibly by 30% or more if the blood supply is poor – as occurs after radiotherapy.

The commonest integrateable implants are Hydroxyapatite and Medpor. These have a variably rough surface and do cause a tissue reaction. Blood vessels and fibroblasts grow into at least their superficial surface. This response may lead to granuloma formation and exposure of the implant. If the implant does become vascularised and integrated it will not extrude and a peg can be inserted by drilling or screwing which will improve motility of the artificial eye.

The simplest and usually cheapest nonintegrateable implant remains an acrylic ball. It is inert but can extrude. An enormous number of other implants have been tried.

ENUCLEATION WITH PRIMARY IMPLANT
(Fig 11.3)

Principle
Complete excision of the eye and insertion of an orbital implant.

Indications
Blind painful eye, intraocular tumour, trauma, risk of sympathetic ophthalmitis, cosmesis.

Method
Steps 1–5 as under enucleation (Fig 11.1a, b, c).

6. Open the posterior part of Tenon's capsule by spreading with blunt scissors and exposing fat (Fig 11.3a). Assess the appropriate

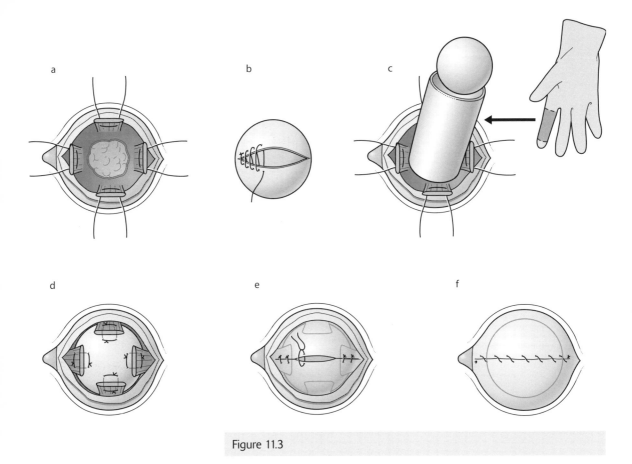

Figure 11.3

size of implant by putting a 'sizer' or sample acrylic implant into this intraconal space i.e. between the rectus muscles. Tenon's capsule must be able to close easily and without tension over the implant. In principle it is desirable to use the largest implant placed as posteriorly as possible.

7. Cover the chosen implant if appropriate (Fig 11.3b). The rectus muscle and inferior oblique can be sutured directly to a dermis fat graft and possibly to a Medpor implant but most of the other implants need a cover to which the muscles can be sutured. Sclera used to be popular but the risk of slow viruses and HIV infection etc. has led to the use of manufactured materials such as vicryl or mersilene mesh. Autogenous tissue such as fascia lata or temporalis fascia can also be used. Whatever material is chosen it should cover the anterior part of the implant and should leave as little material extending posteriorly as possible as this can cause pain and limit motility. The cover also acts as a barrier to limit extrusion.

8. Insert the prepared implant into the cavity using a 'glide' through which it can be slid into place without dragging the orbital

tissues inwards. When the 'glide' is removed the orbital tissues will be everted a little which will help to retain the implant and reduce any tendency to extrusion which can occur by tissue restitution if the wound edges have been inverted. Various 'glides' are available but one of the simplest and cheapest is to cut a finger off a nonstick disposable glove (Fig 11.3c). If the blind end is also cut off this finger, this leaves a nonstick flexible cylinder through which the implant can be nicely directed into the posterior orbit (Fig. 11.3c).

9. Suture the rectus muscles to the implant or cover (Fig 11.3d).
   Note: If the inferior oblique has been saved and can be sutured to the implant or cover it will help to support the implant.
10. Close Tenon's capsule with multiple interrupted 4 '0' long-acting absorbable sutures (Fig 11.3e).
11. Close the conjunctiva with 6 '0' long-acting absorbable running or interrupted sutures and insert a light shell which helps to maintain the fornices but does not press on the suture line (Fig 11.3f).
12. Give systemic antibiotics. Keep double padded for 48 hours, then use antibiotic drops regularly.
13. The wound should be well healed before the socket is moulded and a definitive prosthesis is tried. This may take six weeks.
14. It usually takes about nine months for an integrateable implant to become sufficiently vascularised to consider drilling to insert a peg or to consider screwing in a post to try and improve motility of the artificial eye.

Complications

Pain, infection, wound dehiscence, implant extrusion, granuloma formation.

Most of these can be avoided by attention to the points detailed above. Postoperative anaesthesia can be supplemented by giving an injection of a long-acting local anaesthetic behind the implant at the end of surgery.

If an early wound dehiscence or granuloma formation is detected it may be possible to excise and cauterise the granuloma and resuture the wound. The flaps will need to be undermined extensively enough to allow them to be closed without any tension. If an integrateable implant has been used it may be possible to reduce its size either by burring down the surface with a drill or reducing it with a knife. A barrier material such as fascia lata can be inserted over the implant. The surgery required to be effective is usually much more extensive than anticipated and it is wise to have full anaesthesia facilities available.

If the dehiscence over the implant has been present for some weeks conjunctiva is likely to have grown around the implant which requires removal with its cystic capsule. It can be replaced at the same time with a dermis fat graft or the socket can be allowed to heal and a secondary implant inserted later.

a

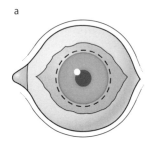

b

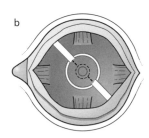

c

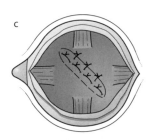

d

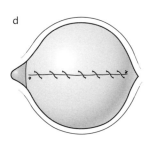

Figure 11.4

EVISCERATION WITH PRIMARY IMPLANT
(Fig 11.4)

Principle

The ocular contents are removed leaving the scleral envelope with its attached extraocular muscles. The sclera is divided. An implant is inserted into the orbital fat and the flaps of sclera are closed over the front of the implant.

Indications

An alternative to enucleation with implant with possibly better cosmesis. Retention of patient's own sclera maximises the mobility of the artificial eye and minimises the risk of extrusion of the implant. *Note*:

1. Intraocular tumours must be excluded as much as possible with ultrasound if appropriate.
2. There is a potential risk of inducing sympathetic ophthalmitis with an evisceration. If a patient has previously had an ocular perforating injury it is wisest to avoid an evisceration.

Method

1. Make a 360° limbal incision through the conjunctiva and Tenon's capsule and undermine to the rectus muscle insertions (Fig 11.4a).
2. Excise the cornea. Eviscerate the ocular contents and clean out all the uveal remnants (Fig 11.2a,b).
3. Cut the scleral envelope into two halves with blunt straight scissors. Make the incision through the sclera beneath the conjunctiva and Tenon's capsule. Cut between the medial and superior rectus muscles and between the inferior and lateral rectus muscles stopping at the optic nerve (Fig 11.4b). Alternatively, similar cuts can be made between the medial and inferior rectus muscles and between the superior and lateral rectus muscles.
4. Cut through the sclera around the optic nerve head to release it and free the two halves of sclera.
5. Assess the appropriate size of implant with a 'sizer' or sample implant and ensure that two halves of sclera with their extraocular muscle attachment can overlap comfortably over the implant.
6. Insert the chosen implant, overlap the edges of the sclera and suture the overlapped sclera with a double row of 5 '0' long-acting absorbable sutures (Fig 11.4c).
7. Close Tenon's capsule and conjunctiva with 6 '0' long-acting absorbable sutures and place a shell to maintain the conjunctival fornices (Fig 11.4d).
8. Give systemic antibiotics, keep padded for 48 hours and then start regular antibiotic drops.

Complications

These are the same as described for enucleation and primary implant. As after any evisceration the potential for causing sympathetic ophthalmitis is not excluded.

POSTENUCLEATION SOCKET SYNDROME (Fig 11.5)

FEATURES

- Enophthalmos
- Deep upper lid sulcus
- Ptosis or lid retraction
- Lax lower lid
- Shallow lower fornix

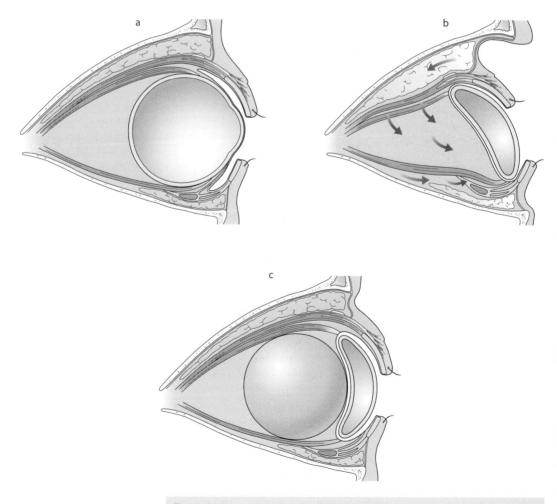

Figure 11.5

When an eye is removed and an orbital implant is not inserted, the subsequent volume deficit causes enophthalmos and a deep upper lid sulcus. The eye is no longer there to support the superior rectus and levator muscle complex which drops to a variable degree, giving rise to ptosis or, more rarely, lid retraction. Lid retraction probably occurs due to the disinserted superior rectus muscle contracting and pulling on the levator complex via the common sheath. The inferior rectus muscle is no longer pushed down by the presence of the eye and it tends to rise in the socket. The inferior fornix becomes shallow due to the associated elevation of the lower lid retractors and their connections. The fat within the orbit tends to collect inferiorly with gravity. There is a related posterior and anticlockwise rotation of the orbital content which may be related to the lower lid fat being held relatively anteriorly by the attachments of the orbital septae, inferior oblique muscle and inferior orbital septum (Fig 11.5a,b).

If a small artificial eye is inserted into a postenucleation socket with no implant, the upper part of the eye tends to tilt backwards and the enophthalmos and deep upper lid sulcus with the ptosis and lid retraction is obvious. If the artificial eye is increased in size it initially improves these features but the lower lid sags under the weight of the artificial eye giving the appearance of a socket which is lower than the other side or a 'dropped socket appearance'. The artificial eye becomes unstable due to the lax lower lid and shallow lower fornix. These features of the postenucleation socket syndrome can be mainly avoided if a suitable sized implant is inserted at the time of an enucleation. If the syndrome is established it can be treated by inserting a secondary orbital implant (Fig 11.5c) and further orbital volume enhancement if necessary as well as correcting the other features of the condition as appropriate.

Management
1. Orbital volume replacement
   a. Secondary implant (intraconal) (Figs 11.5c, 11.6)
   b. Orbital floor implant (Fig 11.7)
   c. Dermis fat graft to upper sulcus (Fig 11.9)
2. Lower lid tightening
   a. Lateral canthal sling
   b. Medial canthal reconstruction
   c. Fascial sling
3. Correction of shallow lower fornix
   a. Fornix deepening sutures
4. Ptosis correction.

SYSTEM FOR POSTENUCLEATION SOCKET SYNDROME

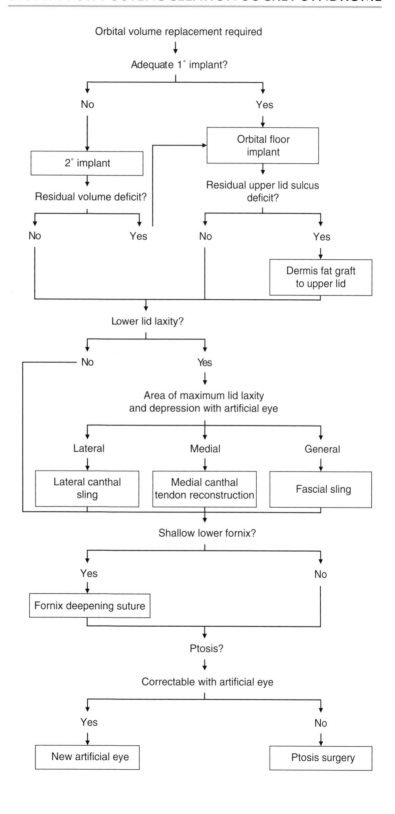

I. ORBITAL VOLUME REPLACEMENT

A. SECONDARY ORBITAL IMPLANT (INTRACONAL) (Fig 11.6)

Principle

The insertion of an orbital implant into the intraconal space i.e. between the extraocular muscles. In a postevisceration socket the sclera can be opened and the implant similarly positioned into the intraconal space.

Indications

To correct an orbital volume deficit if there is no primary implant, an implant with an inadequate volume which needs to be exchanged for a larger implant, or a volume deficit following extrusion of a primary implant.

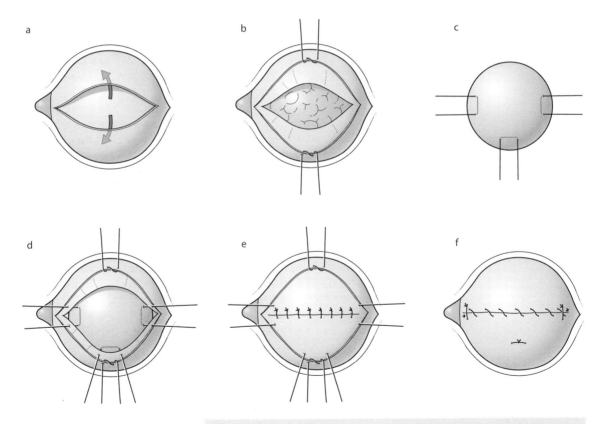

Figure 11.6

Method

1. Preoperatively assess the position of the rectus muscles in the socket by getting the patient to look in different directions. At operation, make a horizontal conjunctival incision above the inferior rectus and below the superior rectus.
2. Separate the conjunctiva from the underlying Tenon's capsule and fibrous tissue. Undermine it extensively both superiorly and inferiorly into the fornices, taking care to stay superficial and not to cut the aponeurosis (Fig.11.6a).
3. Put a traction suture in each conjunctival flap and clip it to the sterile towels.
4. Palpate the socket and make a horizontal cut with scissors through the subconjunctival fibrous tissue towards the apex of the orbit, trying to stay above the inferior rectus. Spread the scissors until intraconal fat is seen (Fig. 11.6b). Remove any previously placed inadequate implant. If there is a postevisceration scleral remnant present, identify the rectus muscles and pass a 4 '0' black silk suture under each one. Use a knife to divide the sclera usually into four segments each with its own rectus muscle and proceed as with an evisceration and primary implant – Stages 4–8.

   Note: After primary evisceration if an implant is to be inserted the sclera is usually divided into two halves. If however a scleral remnant is found when carrying out a secondary implant, the sclera is usually very contracted and it is more easily opened if it is divided into four portions each with its own rectus muscle insertion.

5. In a postenucleation socket pass a traction suture into each of the two fibrous tissue flaps. They contain what remains of Tenon's capsule and the rectus muscle insertions and should impart some movement to the implant.
6. Use a 'sizer' or sample acrylic implant to assess the appropriate size of implant required – usually a 20 or 22 mm diameter ball or integrateable implant or a 25 mm diameter dermis fat graft – and check that the fibrous tissue flaps will close over it easily without tension. If necessary, open the wound further by spreading with blunt scissors.
7. Cover the implant if desired as for a primary implant and insert three double armed 5 '0' long-acting absorbable sutures into the cover or implant itself medially, laterally and inferiorly (Fig 11.6c).
8. Insert the implant into the intraconal fat with a 'glide' as for stage 8 of enucleation with primary implant. Pass the three long-acting absorbable sutures through the fibrous tissue flaps (Fig 11.6d). Close the fibrous tissue flaps with multiple interrupted 4 '0' long-acting absorbable sutures (Fig 11.6e). If a dermis fat graft has been used the graft can either be buried completely under the fibrous tissue flaps or the flaps with the conjunctiva can be sutured to the anterior surface of the graft which is then left bare to granulate.

9. Pass the long-acting absorbable sutures through the conjunctiva. Tie them and close the conjunctiva (Fig 11.6f).

10. The subsequent management is the same as for enucleation with primary implant stages 11–14.

Complications

Same as for a primary implant.

B. ORBITAL FLOOR IMPLANT (Figs 11.7 and 11.8)

Principle

The periosteum of the orbital rim is exposed by (1) a full thickness lateral canthal and conjunctival approach or (2) via skin muscle blepharoplasty flap. The periosteum is elevated and an implant placed subperiostally. The lateral canthal approach allows the lower lid to be tightened and raised laterally by shortening and reattaching the lateral tarsus or lateral canthal tendon to the periosteum of the lateral orbital wall as desired. Orbital floor implants may be:

AUTOGENOUS

– e.g. bone grafts

NONAUTOGENOUS

– Integrateable e.g. Medpor
– Nonintegrateable e.g. Silicone.

Indications

1. Orbital volume enhancement e.g. when an adequate primary or secondary orbital implant is in position. A nonautogenous graft is preferable as it will not absorb.

2. Repair of an orbital floor fracture. An autogenous graft is preferable if the implant is exposed in the antrum or if there is an increased risk of infection, but an integrateable implant can be used.

LATERAL CANTHAL APPROACH (SWINGING EYELID FLAP) (Fig 11.7)

Method

1. Make a full thickness incision at the lateral canthus with scissors and cut down to the orbital rim (Fig 11.7a).

2. Cut through the conjunctiva and lower lid retractors immediately below the tarsus (Fig 11.7b).

3. Open the plane between the preseptal orbicularis muscle and the inferior orbital septum to expose the orbital rim (Fig 11.7c).

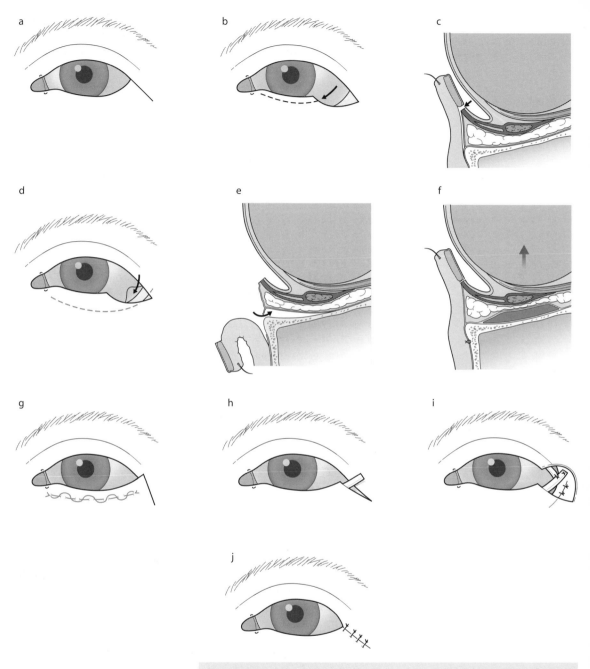

Figure 11.7

4. Cut through the periosteum on the anterior part of the orbital rim and raise an edge of periosteum inferiorly over the maxilla (Fig 11.7d).

5. Elevate the periosteum superiorly over the orbital rim and continue to elevate it over the orbital floor. Identify any orbital floor and associated fractures and elevate any incarcerated orbital contents (Fig 11.7e).

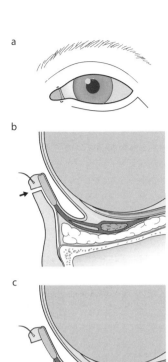

a

b

c

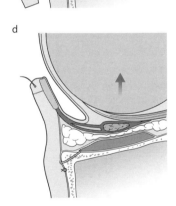

d

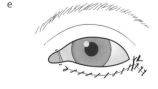

e

Figure 11.8

6. Prepare an appropriate size and type of implant. Use periosteal elevators to elevate the periosteum. Insert the implant under the periosteum. Try to position it posterior to the orbital rim.

   Note: Bone grafts and sheets of integrateable material such as Medpor can be stacked together to try and obtain the optimum volume replacement. A thin silastic sheet may be all that is required for repair of an orbital fracture without a volume deficit. Various preformed orbital implant shapes are available and silicone blocks can be cut to the desired size

7. Try to suture the periosteum together over the implant using 4 '0' long-acting absorbable sutures. If the periosteum is healthy and closes without undue tension it is usually unnecessary to fix the implant more securely (Fig 11.7f). Bulky or unstable implants can be sutured or wired through burr holes in the orbital rim (see Fig 11.8d).

8. Close the conjunctiva with a running 6 '0' long-acting absorbable suture (Fig 11.7g).

9. Close the lateral canthal incision in layers with a direct suture to the intact upper limb of the lateral canthal tendon or, depending on how much tightening is required, with a lateral canthal suture from the lateral tarsus to the periosteum of the lateral orbital rim (p 61) or with a lateral tarsal strip (p 62) (Fig 11.7h,i,j) according to how much lid tightening is required. Whatever technique is used it is wise to leave the lateral canthus supported a little higher than it was preoperatively.

10. Give systemic antibiotics. If treating the postenucleation socket syndrome place a shell behind the eyelids and leave padded for 48 hours before starting antibiotic drops. If treating a patient with a sighted eye monitor the vision as detailed below.

SKIN/MUSCLE BLEPHAROPLASTY APPROACH
(Fig 11.8)

Method

1. Make a subciliary skin incision (Fig 11.8a).
2. Leave a small strip of pretarsal orbicularis muscle close to the lid margin and incise through the orbicularis to expose the tarsus (Fig 11.8b).
3. Dissect anterior to the orbital septum to expose the orbital rim (Fig 11.8c).
4. Proceed as for the lateral canthal approach to the orbital floor stages 4–7 (Fig 11.8d).
5. Support the lid laterally by closing the cut orbicularis with a buried 6 '0' long-acting absorbable suture.
6. Elevate the lateral canthal angle with a 5 '0' black silk suture passed from the skin through the orbicularis muscle into periosteum above the lateral canthus and out through orbicularis muscle and skin.

7. Close the skin flap with a running 6 '0' nylon suture (Fig 11.8e).

8. Remove the sutures at 5 days. Give systemic antibiotics and manage as for the lateral canthal approach.

Complications

Loss of sight, squint, anaesthesia or sensory changes in the infra-orbital nerve distribution, implant extrusion or infection, over- and undercorrection.

These complications can occur with any orbital floor implant. If an orbital floor implant is inserted under a seeing eye there is always the risk of damage to vision and of causing a squint. It is wise to check in the immediate postoperative period in the recovery room that the patient can see and that the pupil reacts. These observations need to be repeated subsequently on the ward. If the patient cannot see the implant should be removed immediately. Any change in ocular position can lead to a squint which may recover spontaneously or require squint surgery. A change in sensation of the maxillary division of the 5th nerve is common but usually recovers. Any implant can become infected or extrude but the risks are reduced if the patient is given systemic antibiotics.

C. DERMIS FAT GRAFT TO UPPER LID (Fig 11.9)

Principle

The superior orbital rim periosteum is exposed via a skin crease incision. A dermis fat graft is harvested, usually from the left lower abdomen (p 26), and the dermis sutured to the periosteum.

Indications

A deep superior sulcus e.g. after trauma in a patient with an eye present or in the postenucleation socket after an adequate intraconal orbital implant and orbital floor implant.

Method

1. Expose the orbital rim via an anterior approach skin crease incision as for a levator resection (p 99) and free any adhesions (Fig 11.9a).

2. Suture the dermis of the graft to the periosteum of the orbital rim with 6 '0' long-acting absorbable sutures. It is usually possible to place one suture posterior to the rim and three along the rim. The fat should fill the preaponeurotic space behind the preseptal orbicularis muscle. Aim to overcorrect the volume deficit by an arbitrary 30% and trim off any excess fat (Fig 11.9b).

3. Advance the levator complex if necessary to correct any ptosis and reform the skin crease with 6 '0' long-acting absorbable sutures which pick up the underlying upper lid retractor.

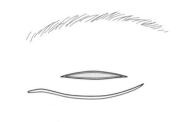
a

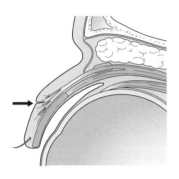

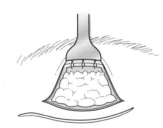
b

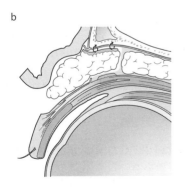

Figure 11.9

Complications

Over correction, under correction, cyst formation, an avascular fat necrosis and fat liquefaction.

Relatively little fat is required to fill an upper lid sulcus and any excess may need to be reduced surgically. Any dermis fat graft may contain epidermal derivatives which may produce cysts which can be excised or hair growth which can be treated with cryotherapy. These complications are rare with upper sulcus dermis fat grafts. In avascular situations such as a postirradiation socket, the fat may liquefy and escape through the upper lid skin crease. Antibiotics are usually given until the discharge stops but the volume of the graft may be excessively reduced.

II. LOWER LID TIGHTENING PROCEDURES

If despite fully correcting the orbital volume deficit as described above, the lower lid is still pushed down by the artificial eye tighten the lid in the area of maximum laxity.

a. Lateral – lateral tarsal strip
b. Medial – medial canthal tendon reconstruction
c. General – fascial sling.

A. LATERAL TARSAL STRIP (See Figs 4.5, 11.7)

Principle

The lower limb of the lateral canthal tendon is cut. The lid is shortened by creating a new lateral canthal tendon from the tarsal plate. This is sutured to the periosteum of the lateral orbital wall at a higher level to compensate for the weight of the artificial eye which will depress the lower lid.

Indications

Lateral canthal laxity. It can be associated with an orbital floor implant.

Method

See ectropion chapter (p 62, Fig 4.5) and orbital floor implant via lateral canthal approach (p 214) (Fig 11.7).

B. MEDIAL CANTHAL TENDON RECONSTRUCTION

Principle

Medial canthal laxity when an artificial eye is present is treated by a full thickness pentagonal resection of the lax area and reformation of the anterior limb of the medial canthal tendon. It is not necessary to reform the posterior limb of the medial canthal tendon as it does not provide a strong enough support for the artificial eye or help to control epiphora.

Indications

Medial canthal laxity.

Method

1. Cut through the full thickness of the lid in the area of maximum laxity.
2. Overlap the edges of the lid margin and resect an appropriate amount of lid or medial canthal tissues.
3. Open (marsupialise) the cut inferior canaliculus.
4. Reform the anterior limb of the medial canthal tendon preferably with a permanent suture such as 4 '0' prolene although a long-acting absorbable suture can be used.
5. Close the lid in layers.

C. FASCIAL SLING (Fig 11.10)

Principle

A strip of fascia is passed through the lid between the medial canthal tendon and the lateral orbital wall.

Indications

Generalised and recurrent lid laxity; need to support a heavy artificial eye.

Method

1. Make a small vertical incision over the medial canthal tendon.
2. Thread both ends of a small length of wire into the eye of a curved needle and pass it under the medial canthal tendon medially where the lacrimal sac is not at risk. Leave a loop of wire exposed to pull the fascia under the tendon (Fig 11.10a).
3. Make a small horizontal incision over the lateral orbital rim lateral to the canthus.
4. Expose the periosteum over the lateral orbital rim.
5. Make a small subciliary incision in the centre of the lower eyelid and cut down to the tarsal plate.
6. Split a 2–3 mm wide strip of fascia along the line of the collagen fibres. Stored or fresh autogenous fascia lata may be used. For details of how to take autogenous fascia lata, see p 24.

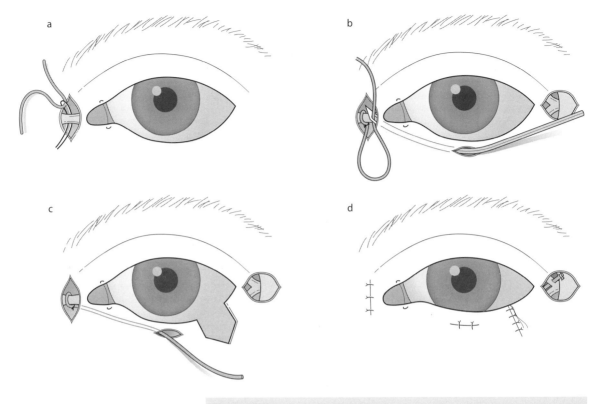

Figure 11.10

7. Use the wire loop to pull one end of the fascial strip through the medial canthal tendon (Fig 11.10a). Suture the fascia to itself with a nonabsorbable suture.

8. Pass a Wright's fascial needle through the central eyelid incision and push it through the lid to the medial canthal incision, keeping deep to the orbicularis muscle, superficial to the tarsal plate, and as near to the lid margin as possible (Fig 11.10b).

9. Withdraw the needle with the fascia and leave it emerging from the central lid incision.

10. If the eyelid is lax, do a full-thickness resection of the lid just lateral to the central eyelid incision; otherwise there will be a tendency for an ectropion when the sling is tightened (Fig 11.10c). Alternatively this resection can be carried out at the lateral canthus.

11. Introduce the needle into the lateral incision, pass through the posterosuperior part of the lateral canthal tendon or through the periosteum of the lateral orbital rim and keeping close to the lid margin bring the needle out through the central lid incision.

12. Withdraw the strip of fascia through the lateral incision.

Note: the fascia can be pulled through a burr hole in the lateral orbital wall if it is not held posteriorly enough by the lateral canthal tendon or periosteum of the lateral orbital rim.

13. Suture it to the periosteum under reasonable tension with a 4 '0' or 5 '0' prolene suture (Fig 11.10d).
14. Close the skin incision with interrupted sutures.

Complications

Foreign body reaction with permanent sutures, lateral ectropion with fascial sling, exposure of sling material.

III. CORRECTION OF SHALLOW LOWER FORNIX

FORNIX DEEPENING SUTURES (Fig 11.11)

Principle

The fornix is created by a silicone rod or gutter held in place with sutures which pass through the periosteum of the orbital rim and are tied on the skin.

Indications

To deepen or reform a shallow fornix where there is no shortage of conjunctiva and there is an orbital implant in position to depress the inferior rectus muscle and its associated lower lid retractors (Fig 11.11a). Fornix deepening sutures can be inserted at the same time as a lower lid tightening procedure if required.

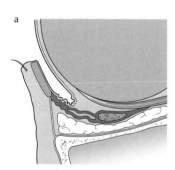

Method

1. Cut approximately a 3 cm long strip of 20 gauge silicone gutter, silicone rod or similar material.
2. Pass both needles of a double-armed 4 '0' prolene suture through the silicone gutter or around a silicone rod etc.
3. Take each needle in turn in a general purpose needle holder, pass it through the conjunctiva of the inferior fornix where the lower fornix should be, engage the surgical periosteum of the orbital rim and exit through the skin of the lower lid and cheek.
4. Place two or more similar sutures and pull the silicone gutter or rod into the fornix. Tie the sutures gently over bolsters on the skin leaving room for tissue swelling (Fig 11.11b). Place a light shell between the lids.

    Note: If there is not enough conjunctiva to reform the fornix without creating an entropion, a mucous membrane graft is required (p 224).

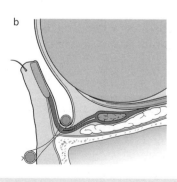

Figure 11.11

5. Leave the sutures for 2–3 weeks or longer unless the bolsters start to cut into the skin, when they should be removed. A shell must be worn continuously to maintain the fornices once the sutures are removed.

Complications

Skin suture marks. The sutures should be tied relatively loosely to prevent this complication and if it starts to occur the suture should be removed early.

IV. PTOSIS CORRECTION

Ptosis should be evaluated after any volume replacement and lower lid surgery has been performed. The prosthesis should be checked first and adjusted to give the best fulcrum effect for the action of the levator muscle. Any residual ptosis can be corrected, based mainly on the levator function as described in Chapter 5.

CONTRACTED SOCKET

A contracted socket may be congenital, e.g. associated with microphthalmos, cystic ocular remnants, anophthalmos, etc., or acquired, e.g. due to trauma, inflammation, radiotherapy, etc. Mild degrees of contraction may cause an entropion or shallow fornices, but in severe cases an artificial eye cannot be retained. Socket expansion is usually possible with the use of special expanders and conformers in congenital cases and with grafts in acquired cases. If the socket is moist these are mucous membrane grafts and if the socket is dry skin grafts are used. If there is a volume deficit in addition to the contracted socket and shortage of lining, a dermis fat graft can be inserted and its surface left bare to conjunctivalise. Alternatively an orbital implant can be buried under whatever vascularised tissue can be found and a graft added to increase the lining. If the socket is very contracted the blood supply is often very poor, e.g. after irradiation, and vascularised tissue may need to be brought into the socket such as a temporalis muscle flap. These techniques are beyond the scope of this book.

I. CONGENITAL

ANOPHTHALMOS/MICROPHTHALMOS AND CONGENITAL SMALL SOCKET

Children born without an eye or with a microphthalmic eye with a diameter of less than 15 mm have a congenital small socket and eyelids. It is essential to try to stretch the tissues with expanders starting as young as possible. Socket conformers of increasing size can be used but their insertion into the conjunctival sac may cause damage and increase fibrosis. Hydrophilic shapes have been developed which can be inserted into the conjunctival sac and as they take up tears they expand, gently increasing the size of the socket. The expansion can then be continued with conventional conformers, shapes and artificial eyes. The conjunctival sac often expands reasonably well but the eyelids may remain small with a ring of peripalpebral fibrosis which is difficult to overcome without surgery. Balloon expanders can be buried within the bony orbit and when inflated can increase the orbital dimensions considerably. Once the child is older expanders are unlikely to help and further treatment will involve increasing the bony socket with bone grafts, screws and plates and building up the eyelids with reconstructive techniques and mucous membrane grafts etc.

II. ACQUIRED

SYSTEM FOR ACQUIRED CONTRACTED SOCKET

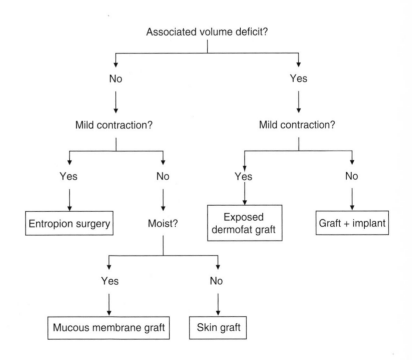

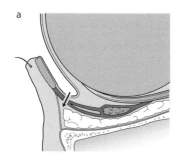

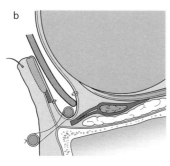

Figure 11.12

MANAGEMENT OF MILD SOCKET CONTRACTION

Entropion surgery

- Upper lid entropion: anterior lamella repositioning ± grey-line split (see p 42)
- Lower lid entropion: grey-line split and retractor repositioning (see p 40).

MANAGEMENT OF MORE SEVERE SOCKET CONTRACTION

- Moist: mucous membrane graft
- Dry: skin graft

FORNIX DEEPENING SUTURES AND MUCOUS MEMBRANE GRAFT (Fig 11.12)

Principle

The most important area to expand in the contracted socket is the fornices. If the socket is moist a mucous membrane graft is taken from the mouth and used to increase the lining of the relevant contracted socket fornix or fornices. The graft is held against the orbital rim with a silicone rod or gutter and sutures.

Indications

Contracted conjunctival fornices which are moist. The technique can be used for either an upper or lower fornix or both and is the same if an eye is present e.g. after chemical trauma.

Method

1. Make an incision through the scarred conjunctiva in the upper and/or lower fornix (Fig 11.12a). Try to leave some conjunctiva at the apex of the socket to which the graft can be sutured.
2. Free and if necessary excise scar tissue to create an adequate defect. *Note*: If this dissection in an upper fornix involves a risk to the levator muscle, it is wise to isolate the muscle first via a skin crease incision through the lid.
3. Suture the mucous membrane graft to the edges of the defect with a 6 '0' continuous absorbable suture.
4. Hold the graft in place with fornix deepening sutures (p 221), which pass through the mucous membrane grafts. In the upper fornix these sutures are passed on either side of the levator complex and out through the superior orbital rim periosteum. In the lower fornix they are positioned as desired.
5. If the levator complex has been exposed through a skin crease incision carry out an upper lid entropion correction of the anterior lamella repositioning type with or without a grey-line split.

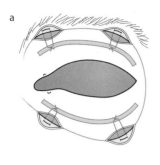

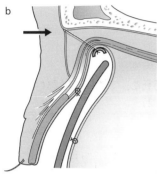

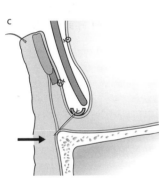

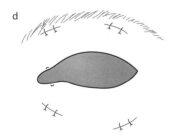

Figure 11.13

6. Tighten the fornix deepening sutures very gently to hold the grafts against their bed but allow for some postoperative swelling. Tie the sutures over bolsters or through a silicone gutter on the skin. Place a shell conformer between the lids (or a ring conformer if an eye is present) (Fig 11.12b).

7. Leave the sutures for between 2 and 4 weeks. They will create skin problems if they are left for more than 4 weeks. If it is desirable to maintain the fornix deepening sutures and pressure on the grafts for longer than 4 weeks, the sutures must be tied in the fornices and not on the skin (as described below).

Complications

Skin suture marks if sutures left for more than 4 weeks or sutures tied too tightly. Infection, granuloma formation at host graft junction.

SOCKET RECONSTRUCTION WITH MUCOSAL GRAFTS (Fig 11.13)

Principle

The fornix or socket lining deficit is expanded with mucous membrane grafts if the socket is moist or skin grafts if the socket is dry. A silicone rod or gutter is sutured to the periosteum of the orbital rim to maintain pressure on the graft for preferably more than 12 weeks i.e. long enough to overcome the phase of fibrous tissue contraction. The sutures are tied over the silicone rod or gutter within the socket and hence do not cause problems with the skin.

Indications

Socket and fornix expansion when there is marked contraction and fibrosis rather than merely a deficiency of the conjunctiva. Such major fornix and socket contraction may be recurrent e.g. after chronic infection, chemical burns, irradiation etc.

Method

Steps 1–3 as for Fornix deepening sutures and mucous membrane graft (p 224).

4. Make 2–4 stab incisions through the skin and orbicularis down to the orbital rim.

5. Pass 4 '0' nylon or prolene sutures through the graft, through the periosteum of the orbital rim, and out through the stab incision. Then re-enter the stab incision, pick up the periosteum again and pass back through the graft.

6. Repeat this with a different suture through each stab incision. In the upper lid if the levator complex has been exposed through a skin crease incision it may be easier to expose the orbital rim

periosteum and pass the suture into it under direct vision. Avoid passing the sutures through the levator complex.

7. Pass the sutures through a silicone gutter, around a silicone rod, or through a conformer that holds the graft in its bed and tie them within the socket fornices (Fig 11.13a,b,c).

8. Suture the stab incisions and place a shell between the lids (Fig 11.13d).

9. Keep the lids padded for 48 hours and then start local antibiotic drops every 2 hours.

10. Remove the stab incision skin sutures at 5 days or earlier. The nylon or prolene sutures holding the graft to the orbital rim should be left for as long as possible to overcome fibrosis and contraction. If they become infected they may have to be removed, but otherwise they can be left for many months provided that a shell is worn that prevents the rod or conformer from becoming buried.

Complications

Infection around one or more sutures. Treatment: Remove the relevant suture and give systemic antibiotics.

SOCKET RECONSTRUCTION WITH SKIN GRAFTS

Principle

The lining of a contracted dry socket is enlarged with skin grafts.

Indications

A contracted dry socket or one in which there is a mixture of skin and conjunctiva or mucous membrane. This causes irritation, desquamation and a foul smelling discharge. All mucosal elements must therefore be removed if the socket is to be reconstructed with skin. Thick split thickness skin is usually preferable to full thickness skin.

Method

The same techniques can be used as with mucous membrane grafts for keeping the skin grafts again the orbital rim.

If the contraction is very severe an attempt may be made at reconstruction by widely opening the socket and excising all previous lining and scar tissue. Split skin is wrapped around a conformer with the raw surface peripheral. The conformer is buried in the socket and the lid remnants sutured together over it. If this is left for long enough it is sometimes possible to create some form of socket.

Complications

Foul smelling discharge if conjunctival or mucosal remnants and skin grafts are present in the same socket.

CONTRACTED SOCKET WITH ASSOCIATED VOLUME DEFICIT

Management of:
- Mild contraction: Exposed dermis fat graft
- Severe contraction: Mucous membrane or skin graft and buried orbital implant

DERMIS FAT GRAFT

Principle

A dermis fat graft is inserted into a volume deficient and lining deficient socket. The anterior surface of the dermis fat graft is left bare to conjunctivalise so that there is a gain in both lining and volume.

Indications

A moderately contracted moist socket with a volume deficit.

Method

1. Make a horizontal incision through the conjunctiva and deeper tissues of the moderately contracted socket.
2. Open the deeper tissues to expose orbital fat between the rectus muscles and stretch this space with a 'sizer' or acrylic implant.
3. Take a suitably sized dermis fat graft which has been harvested as described on p 26 and insert this into the exposed space.
4. Suture the deep tissues of the socket to the edges of the dermis fat graft and try to suture the conjunctiva onto the anterior dermal surface with 6 '0' long-acting absorbable sutures. Leave a bare area of dermis to conjunctivalise.
5. Place a light conformer to maintain the fornices. Leave padded for 48 hours, then start antibiotic drops.
   Note: The exposed dermis will be very white initially but will gradually conjunctivalise and become pink. There will be a gain in both orbital contents and lining making this a valuable technique in the contracted socket.

Complications

As with any dermis fat graft the fat may necrose and liquefy, leading to a divet which can be excised at a later date if required. Hair growth and cyst formation can also occur and can be treated with cryotherapy and excision of the cyst respectively.

ORBITAL IMPLANT AND GRAFT

Principle

An orbital implant is inserted posteriorly into the posterior socket to increase the orbital volume. It is buried under whatever tissue is available or can be brought into the socket as vascular tissue. The lining of the socket is increased with a graft of mucous membrane if the socket is moist and of skin if the socket is dry.

Indications

Very contracted and volume deficient socket.

Method

1. Follow secondary orbital implant (p 212).
   Note: An autogenous or any nonautogenous implant can be used but the size is usually reduced due to scarring of the fibrous tissue flaps.
2. Follow fornix deepening sutures and mucous membrane graft or socket reconstruction with mucosal or skin grafts as described above.
   Note: If the contracted socket is very avascular e.g. after irradiation, vascularised tissue may need to be brought into the socket e.g. a flap of temporalis muscle, a free vascularised pedicle flap, a frontalis muscle, periosteal or midline forehead flap. These techniques are beyond the scope of this book.

Complications

Extrusion of implant. Recurrent contraction.

Cosmetic surgery

12

- Assessment
- Examination
- Consultation/Management

ASSESSMENT

PRESENTING COMPLAINT

Ask the patient what they dislike and want changed, removed or reduced. Give them a mirror and ask them to show you their 'problem'. Look at any photographs from when the patient was younger which might help to demonstrate the changes and show what the patient wants to improve.

HISTORY

Check how long they have had the problem and if there has been any recent change which might indicate a medical condition such as thyroid problems. Beware of the slow changes which might indicate hypothyroidism. Ask about any general medical problems. Check if the patient is on any medication especially aspirin, nonsteroidal anti-inflammatory drugs or vitamin E. These can all make it difficult to control bleeding at surgery and cause increased postoperative bruising and haematomas.

EXAMINATION

- Periorbital position
- Excess tissue
- Lid level and laxity
- Ophthalmic examination
- Photographic record

PERIORBITAL POSITION

BROW PTOSIS

Measure and record the distance between the upper lid margin and the start of the brow hairs with the eye in the primary position of gaze (see Fig 1.6). This is notoriously inaccurate particularly if the patient plucks their eyebrows. It also varies with the frontalis action, presence of any eyelid ptosis, degree of animation and if the patient has had botulinum toxin injections. The normal range for a middle aged person will be 10–15 mm. If the measurement is less than 10 mm the patient definitely has a brow ptosis.

CHEEK PTOSIS

It is difficult to define measurements for a cheek ptosis but record any indicative signs such as a supramalar sulcus or tear trough deformity, increased nasolabial or nasojugal fold and general depression or sag of the cheek tissues (see Fig 1.9).

EXCESS TISSUE

SKIN

The apparent excess skin in the upper lid is related to:

1. brow position
2. amount of skin
3. skin crease.

The amount of skin in the upper lid can be assessed by pushing up the brow and with the patient looking down measuring the vertical distance between the lowest brow hairs and the lid margin (see Fig 1.5). This measurement is inaccurate but if it is more than 25 mm the excess skin can usually be safely removed. It is unwise to leave less than 20 mm or the patient may develop symptoms of lagophthalmos. The position and definition of the skin crease is important as this holds the excess skin away from the lid margin.

MUSCLE

A 'full' upper lid is usually not due so much to excess muscle as to other tissues such as preaponeurotic or periorbital fat, a relative proptosis etc. In the lower lid orbicularis muscle hypertrophy is very much an entity, particularly in people who play a lot of outdoor sport e.g. tennis and who have not worn sunglasses or a peaked cap etc. It can be assessed by getting the patient to smile or grimace and noting the extent of the pretarsal muscle bulge and rhytides.

FAT

Note any excess in the two preaponeurotic fat pockets in the upper lid and in the three pockets in the lower lid.

The temporal or brow fat pad is part of the periorbital fat which lies in front of the orbital septum and under the orbital orbicularis muscle. It is often enlarged in patients with thyroid problems. The periorbital fat pad thickening may extend throughout the upper eyelid periorbital region.

A lacrimal gland prolapse can present as an apparent upper lid lateral fat pad below the brow fat pad. It is a very mobile rounded swelling and is lower and more lateral than the classical upper lid fat prolapses.

Lower lid fat prolapses can be enhanced by cheek ptosis which gives rise to a supramalar sulcus or tear trough deformity (see Figs 1.9, 1.10). If the arcus marginalis and inferior orbital septum is intact and the cheek drops, the inferior lower lid skin comes to lie almost directly over the orbital rim. This creates the supramalar sulcus or 'owl eye' and dark circle appearance and accentuates any lower lid fat prolapse.

LID LEVEL AND LAXITY

In the upper lid measure and record any degree of eyelid ptosis, the height and depth of the skin crease and the levator function.

In the lower lid record any lower lid retraction, scleral show and the position and degree of any lower lid laxity.

OPHTHALMIC EXAMINATION

Record visual acuity in each eye and carry out a full ophthalmic examination. Note any tendency to blepharoconjunctivitis, meibomitis, dry eye, poor blink, etc.

PHOTOGRAPHIC RECORD

Record and keep a photographic record of the patient's preoperative appearance at least with the patient looking straight ahead and with both eyes closed.

CONSULTATION/MANAGEMENT

Having established what the patient wants changed and having examined the patient, the next stage is to explain as much as possible and show the patient what you think the options are for trying to help them.

BROW LIFT

Give them a mirror and show them the effects of raising the brow to establish whether or not they want a brow lift.

UPPER LID BLEPHAROPLASTY

Show them the excess skin that can be removed and the effect of raising and reforming the skin crease. A bent piece of soft wire such as an unravelled paperclip is very effective for this. Try to establish how much upper lid show they would like (see Fig 1.6). Also, do they want a permanent skin crease or would they prefer as little scar as possible? If they want as little scar as possible will they accept that the pretarsal skin will not be as smooth as it would be if the skin crease was reformed tightening the pretarsal skin but leaving them with more of a scar and a better defined skin crease?

MID FACE LIFT

Show the patient the effect of pushing up the cheek and what this does to the nasolabial and nasojugal fold and to any supramalar sulcus or tear trough deformity. Try to establish whether they want this amount of surgery or whether they would be content with camouflaging any supramalar sulcus by releasing the arcus marginalis and lower orbital septum and mobilising fat over the orbital rim.

LOWER LID BLEPHAROPLASTY

Show the patient how excess skin is removed and where the scar will be. Establish whether they would prefer this approach with the possibility of removing excess skin and muscle or whether they would prefer the conjunctival approach and no scar. Are they interested in having the skin retextured with laser resurfacing? Discuss what can be achieved with lateral canthal surgery and its effect on tightening the lower lid and correcting any lid retraction. Will they accept any elevation of the lateral canthus? How much fat do they want removed or are they happy to have it reduced if necessary and mobilised over the orbital rim?

UPPER LID COSMETIC AND FUNCTIONAL BLEPHAROPLASTY

- Upper lid blepharoplasty
- With supratarsal fixation and skin crease reformation
- With lacrimal gland prolapse

- With aponeurosis advancement
- With Muller's muscle resection

UPPER LID BLEPHAROPLASTY (Fig 12.1)

Principle

Upper lid skin is excised with or without orbicularis muscle and fat.

Indications

Cosmesis; excess skin that is creating a visual field defect or causing discomfort by resting on the eyelashes; need to obtain full thickness skin for a graft.

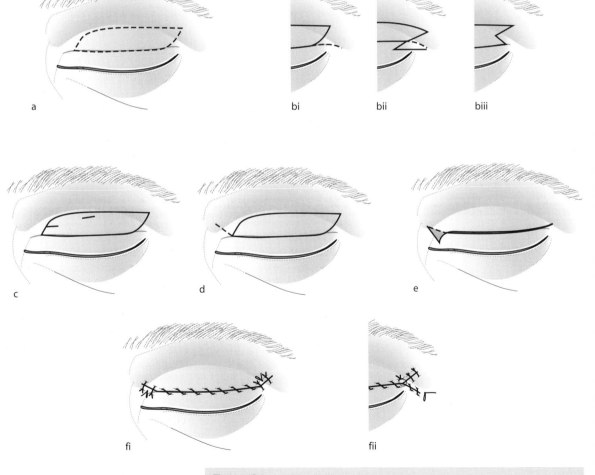

a   bi   bii   biii

c   d   e

fi   fii

Figure 12.1

Method

1. Mark the upper lid skin crease, stopping at the upper punctum.

2. Pick up excess skin, with forceps, based in the skin crease and mark the upper limit that may be excised while still allowing the lids just to meet on gentle closure.

3. At the lateral canthus raise the excision lines towards the brow to prevent hooding (Fig 12.1a). Do not extend into the thick skin beyond the orbital rim as this may produce visible scars (Fig 12.1b).

4. Infiltrate with local anaesthetic, unless the operation is under general anaesthesia, and make the skin incisions, taking care to keep the skin under slight tension.

5. Excise the skin with scissors or use a blade, laser, radio frequency or other cutting and haemostatic instrument to free its connection from the underlying orbicularis muscle.

6. Cauterise any bleeding points.

7. Assess the upper lid bulk which can be caused by preaponeurotic or brow fat and orbicularis muscle. Excise a strip of orbicularis if appropriate.

8. If there is excess preaponeurotic upper lid fat, prolapse it with pressure on the lower lid and push a pair of sharp pointed scissors through the orbital septum into the prolapse. Spread the scissors horizontally, parallel to the aponeurosis, and allow the fat to prolapse through the incision or open the orbital septum completely. The medial fat pad is frequently unsightly and needs reduction. It is paler than the central fat pad. Care should be taken not to remove excess fat from the central fat pad as this can cause alterations in the skin crease (Fig 12.1c).

9. Clamp the prolapsed fat in curved microartery forceps without exerting any traction on the fat pad. Excise the fat above the forceps and cauterise the cut edge. Hold the fat with ordinary forceps and release the artery forceps. Cauterise any vessels that bleed after releasing the artery forceps and allow the fat to retract back into the orbit. It is not necessary to close the orbital septum or orbicularis muscle.

10. If there is excess brow fat undermine under the orbicularis muscle and in front of the orbital septum and periosteum of the superior orbital rim. Reduce this fat extending superiorly and temporally as far as the temporal end of the brow hairs and medially for about the lateral one-third of the upper eyelid just below the lower brow hairs. This extent can be increased subsequently if desired, but beware of the supraorbital nerve.

11. Excise the medial excess skin 'dog ear' as required (Fig 12.1d,e).

12. If there is excess skin laterally (temporal hooding) make an incision in the line of continuation of the skin crease (Fig 12.1bi). Undermine the triangular flap of temporal skin and muscle (Fig 12.1bii). Overlap the skin crease extension line and excise the

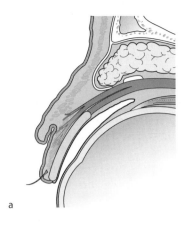

a

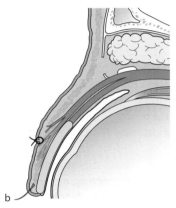

b

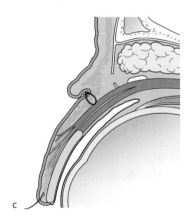

c

Figure 12.2

excess skin and muscle. This creates a 'fish tail' and breaks up the temporal scar (Fig 12.1biii).

13. Close the skin wound with interrupted sutures at the two angulations in the incision. Close the central part of the wound with a continuous suture and used interrupted sutures medially and laterally (Fig 12.1fi). If there is a 'fish tail' laterally close this with an 'apical' suture (Fig 12.1fii). The skin crease can be reformed by closing the skin edges with sutures which pick up the underlying aponeurosis as described below under supratarsal fixation. This creates a more visible scar than by just closing the skin with a continuous suture but the pre-tarsal skin is tightened.

14. Roll the excised skin in a moist gauze swab and keep it in a sterile container in the refrigerator for 3 days. If the eye will not tolerate the amount of skin that has been removed, it can be replaced.

15. Postoperative ice packs may reduce oedema. If fat has been excised it is essential that if any dressing is applied, it can be easily and quickly removed to inspect the pupil. This must be done if the patient complains of discomfort and the vision and pupil must be checked (see below).

16. All sutures should be removed at 5 days.

Complications

Loss of vision. This may occur after any operation in which fat has been removed from the upper or lower eyelids. The cause is thought to be either a deep haemorrhage causing pressure effects on the optic nerve or spasm of vessels supplying the optic nerve. If the pupil begins to dilate and the patient complains of visual loss, the wound must be opened and the orbit decompressed as an emergency to try and prevent possible blindness. If a haematoma is not found and the vision and pupillary signs do not improve, the patient should be vasodilated with drugs such as glyceryl trinitrate to try and overcome any vascular spasm. The intraocular pressure can also be lowered as much as possible to encourage ocular vascular perfusion.

Limitation of eyelid closure from removal of excess skin or the temporary limiting effects of skin crease reformation sutures. Initial treatment is with lubricants and removal of the skin crease sutures. Eyelid closure usually improves with time and massage but if need be skin can be replaced. This is easy if the excised skin has been kept.

Asymmetry of skin crease, upper lid show or skin fold. If this does not settle with time a revision may be necessary.

Scarring. If the scar is thickened and elevated it usually settles with massage and possibly local steroids. If the scar is atrophic and stretches it will need a scar revision with excision of the old scar and better support of the wound with subcutaneous long-acting absorbable sutures.

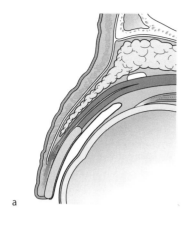

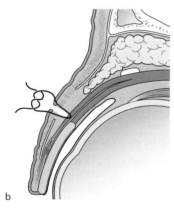

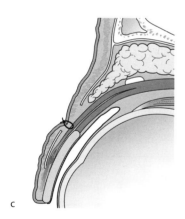

Figure 12.3

SUPRATARSAL FIXATION AND SKIN CREASE REFORMATION (Figs 12.2 12.3)

Principle

Excess upper lid skin is excised in a standard blepharoplasty (Fig 12.2a,b) and 'tucked' in the technique of supratarsal fixation (Fig 12.2c). The skin crease is reformed. It can be raised and excess skin excised.

Indications

A patient requiring a blepharoplasty and skin crease reformation who has a low skin crease, an inadequate tear film or poor lid closure from any cause in whom it is especially desirable not to excise very much skin. Lax pretarsal skin can be smoothed out and put under slight tension by reforming the skin crease.

Method

1. Mark the proposed new skin crease. This should be 10–11 mm above the lid margin for a true supratarsal fixation but for a skin crease reformation it can be anywhere.
2. Inject local anaesthetic, if not under general anaesthesia, and excise the skin as before.
3. Excise a strip of orbicularis muscle to expose the aponeurosis.
4. Open the orbital septum and excise fat if required.
5. Close the skin edges and reform a skin crease with interrupted 6 '0' absorbable sutures that pick up the underlying aponeurosis (Fig 12.2c).

   Note: supratarsal fixation is a variation of the anterior approach skin crease reformation described on (p 106) A similar technique can be used to create a skin crease and 'westernise' Orientals (Fig 12.3). The skin crease can be set at any desired level but it is important to excise subcutaneous fat, orbicularis and preaponeurotic fat to create an effective adhesion between the skin and aponeurosis.

Complications

See Upper lid blepharoplasty.

Fixed skin crease scar which initially limits upgaze, can cause prolonged upper lid oedema and take a long time to settle.

LACRIMAL GLAND PROLAPSE REPAIR (Fig 12.4)

Principle

The superior orbital septum close to the arcus marginalis is sutured to Whitnall's superior suspensory ligament with nonabsorbable

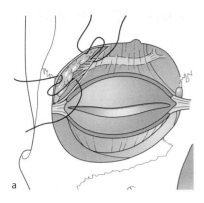

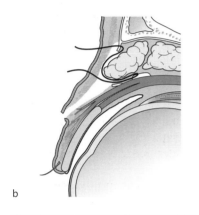

Figure 12.4

sutures (Fig 12.4a,b). This creates a barrier which prevents the lacrimal gland from prolapsing forward.

Indications

Prolapsed lacrimal gland.

Method

Stages 1–10 as for upper lid blepharoplasty.

11. Open the orbital septum fully if this has not already been done. Try to leave about 5 mm of the septum attached to the arcus marginalis.
12. Identify the prolapsed lacrimal gland as a lobulated mass which is paler and firmer tissue than preaponeurotic fat.
13. Expose Whitnall's superior suspensory ligament of the globe.
14. Reposition the gland with a squint hook and suture the edge of the cut orbital septum to Whitnall's ligament with about $3 \times 6/0$ nylon sutures (Fig. 12.4a, b).
15. Continue stages 11–16 for upper lid blepharoplasty.

Complications

Limitation of eyelid closure. This occurs if the sutures are placed into the levator muscle and not into Whitnall's ligament. It usually resolves in time but if it does not the sutures will need to be removed and replaced.

Recurrence of prolapse. Treatment is to repeat the procedure.

UPPER LID BLEPHAROPLASTY AND APONEUROTIC ADVANCEMENT (Fig 12.5)

Principle

Aponeurosis advancement or upper lid retractor shortening is combined with a blepharoplasty (Fig 12.5a,b).

Indications

Frank ptosis and excess upper lid tissue.

Method

Stage 1–10 as for upper lid blepharoplasty.

11. Cut through the thinned aponeurosis with scissors at the original skin crease incision (Fig. 12.5a).
12. Identify and clean the anterior surface of the tarsal plate. Do exactly the same bilaterally even if the ptosis only involves one side.

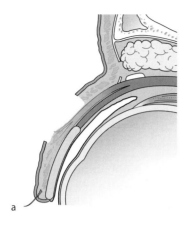

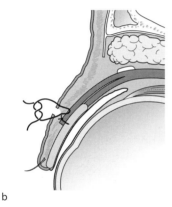

a

b

Figure 12.5

13. If the ptosis is unilateral, suture the aponeurosis of the unaffected side directly to the tarsus with 3 × 6/0 long-acting absorbable sutures.

14. Advance the healthy aponeurosis on the involved side as appropriate to try and set the two lids at approximately the same height and contour. Suture the aponeurosis with 3 × 6/0 long-acting absorbable sutures as on the unaffected side.

15. If there is a significant bilateral ptosis the aponeurosis of both sides can be advanced similarly.

16. Continue as for stages 11–16 of upper lid blepharoplasty and reform the skin crease (Fig. 12.5b).

Complications

Asymmetry. Despite performing surgery on both upper lids at the same time it is remarkably difficult to end up with a symmetrical result and the ptosis fully corrected.

Overcorrection. Manage this with traction and massage etc. exactly as described under aponeurotic ptosis repair (p.99).

BLEPHAROPLASTY AND MÜLLER'S MUSCLE RESECTION (Fig 12.6)

Principle

A blepharoplasty is combined with a Müller's muscle and conjunctival resection (Fig 12.6a,b).

Indications

The patient who does not have a significant ptosis but wants the eyes to look 'bigger' and more 'open' after a blepharoplasty. It is easier to achieve a satisfactory symmetrical result with this technique than by advancing the aponeurosis.

Method

Complete an upper lid blepharoplasty stages 1–13 and then evert the lid.

14. Use two forceps to pick up about 8 mm of conjunctiva and Müller's muscle above the tarsal plate at the medial and lateral extremities of the lid. Stay superficial to avoid picking up the aponeurosis.

15. Replace the forceps with two temporary sutures or apply a Putterman clamp if one is available.

16. Excise the 8 mm of folded conjunctiva and Müller's muscle between the two sutures or held in the clamp and stop any bleeding (Fig. 12.6a).

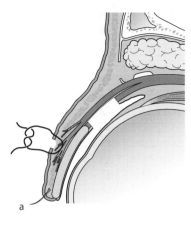

a

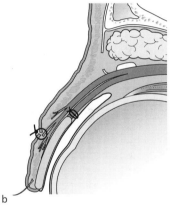

b

Figure 12.6

17. Close the wound with a 7 '0' buried long-acting absorbable suture or a 6 '0' pull-out nylon suture passed through the whole eyelid and removed with the blepharoplasty sutures at five days (Fig. 12.6b).

Complications

As with any posterior approach ptosis surgery the patient can get some corneal irritation or rarely an abrasion.

LOWER LID BLEPHAROPLASTY

- Skin flap
- Skin muscle flap
- Conjunctival approach

SKIN FLAP BLEPHAROPLASTY (Fig 12.7)

Principle

Lower lid skin is excised with or without fat.

Indications

Cosmesis; excess fine skin; excess fat for reduction but not mobilization.

Method

1. Mark the eyelid skin 1–2 mm below the lashes from the lower punctum to the lateral canthus.
2. Continue the line laterally from the lateral canthus staying relatively horizontal but dropping a little (Fig 12.7a).
3. If the patient is not under a general anaesthetic, infiltrate subcutaneously with local anaesthetic and incise the skin, holding it under slight tension.
4. Undermine the flap from the underlying orbicularis muscle and cauterise the bleeding points (Fig 12.7b). As with any blepharoplasty a blade and scissors, laser, radio frequency or any other cutting and haemostasing instrument can be used.
5. If there is excess lower lid fat, prolapse it by pushing on the upper lid. Push a pair of sharp-pointed scissors through the orbicularis muscle and orbital septum into the fat prolapse. Spread the scissors horizontally in the line of the muscle fibres and allow the fat to prolapse. The lateral fat pad is much smaller than the medial one. It should be approached first or it may be difficult to find. Two incisions are usually required for the medial fat pad (Fig 12.7c).
6. Excise and cauterise the fat as for the upper lid – stage 9.

7. Pull the flap over the lid margin with gentle upward and lateral traction. Make a small vertical cut through it down to the estimated position of its new apex. Cut off any vertical excess skin extending above the subciliary incision as a thin triangle with its base laterally at the new apex. When cutting the skin think of it as a long thin rectangle with the medial end triangulated. This will help to avoid taking more skin in the lateral part of the eyelid. Cut off the excess horizontal skin from the same apical point as a lateral triangle with its base upwards (Fig 12.7d).

   Note: a. It is vital not to excise too much skin vertically as this can cause an ectropion. If the operation is under a local anaesthetic, get the patient to look over the top of his head and open his mouth at the same time. With the skin stretched in this way any vertical excess can be safely excised.

   b. If there is excess horizontal laxity of the whole lid that causes it to sag, tighten the lid at the lateral canthus with a lateral canthal suture, a lateral tarsal strip or carry out a full thickness pentagonal lid resection under the blepharoplasty flap as described under involutional ectropion (p 60-63).

8. Suture the lateral angulation of the skin flap into position with an interrupted suture of 5 '0' black silk. This should pick up deep tissue or the periosteum over the orbital rim slightly above the lateral canthus to provide a little elevation and support to the flap. The suture should not be tied tightly or it may bury itself, be difficult to remove and create a depression. Such a deep suture is not required if a lateral canthal tightening procedure has been carried out.

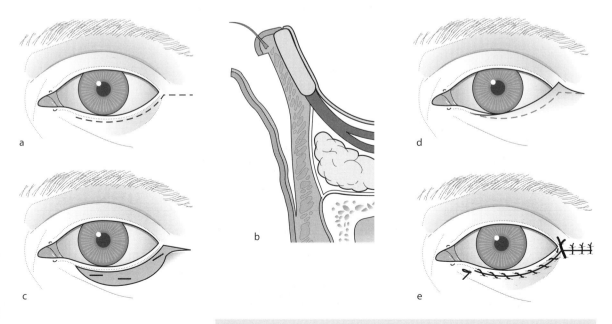

a

b

c

d

e

Figure 12.7

9. Close the subciliary incision with a continuous suture and the lateral incision with interrupted sutures (Fig 12.7e).
10. All sutures should be removed by five days.

Complications

Visual loss. This can occur if fat has been removed. Manage as under upper lid blepharoplasty.

Lower lid retraction and ectropion. This occurs from removal of excess skin or from failure to recognise and treat lid laxity prophylactically or from middle lamella scarring. If it does not correct itself with time and upward massage it may require (1) lower lid tightening or (2) the addition of skin.

Visible scars. Manage as under upper lid blepharoplasty.

SKIN-MUSCLE FLAP BLEPHAROPLASTY (Fig 12.8)

Principle

Lower lid skin and muscle is excised with or without fat.

Indications

Cosmesis; excess skin and muscle, especially if there is orbicularis muscle hypertrophy; excess fat for reduction or mobilization to camouflage a supramalar sulcus and to try to reduce colour changes and 'dark circles' around the lower lids.

Method

Stages 1–3 as for skin flap blepharoplasty (p 239).

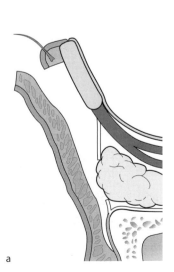
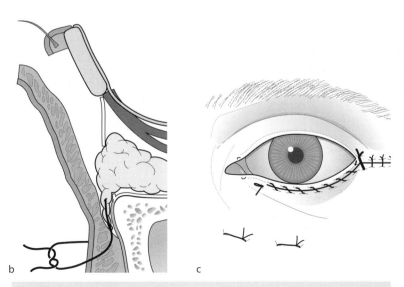

a   b   c

Figure 12.8

4. Cut through the orbicularis muscle in the line of the lateral skin incision to expose the suborbicularis space over the orbital rim.

5. Open this plane in front of the orbital septum with blunt scissors and use them to cut the orbicularis muscle along the subciliary incision.

6. Pull the tarsus upwards with toothed forceps and use blunt dissection to separate the skin-muscle flap from the orbital septum down to the inferior orbital rim.

7. Divide the orbital septum at the arcus marginalis and open the fat capsule to release and mobilise the lower lid fat (Fig 12.8a).

8. Reduce any excess fat by clamping and cutting as described under stage 9 for upper lid blepharoplasty.

9. If there is a supramalar sulcus free the orbicularis muscle from the orbital rim and create a space under the muscle and over the suborbicularis oculi fat. Mobilise the released fat into this space. It can be held in this position if desired with double-armed 4 '0' prolene traction sutures each needle of which is passed through the fat, through the orbicularis and is tied loosely on the skin of the cheek at an appropriate level (Fig 12.8b).

10. Excise the excess skin and muscle from the flap essentially as described for excising skin only with a skip flap blepharoplasty stage 7. If there is orbicularis muscle hypertrophy more orbicularis muscle than skin can be cautiously removed.

11. Suture the lateral angulation of the skin flap as for skin flap blepharoplasty stage 8. The 5 '0' black silk suture should close the cut orbicularis and support the lid. The cut orbicularis should also be closed with a buried 6 '0' long-acting absorbable suture for additional support.

12. The subciliary incision should be closed with a continuous suture and interrupted sutures should be used to close the lateral wound, taking care to evert the wound edges (Fig 12.8c). These sutures and the fat repositioning sutures should be removed by about five days.

Complications

As for lower lid skin flap blepharoplasty.

CONJUNCTIVAL APPROACH (Fig 12.9)

Principle

The lower lid fat is debulked via a conjunctival approach.

Indications

Cosmesis; lower lid fat reduction without any scar on the skin i.e. usually younger patients with fat prolapses and no excess skin or muscle. In addition the lid can be tightened at the lateral canthus. The skin

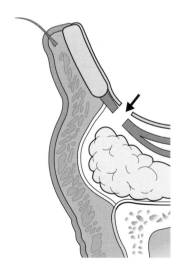

Figure 12.9

can be retextured with laser. The lower lid fat can be mobilised into the supramalar sulcus.

Method

1. If the patient is not under general anaesthesia apply local anaesthetic drops. Infiltrate local anaesthetic subconjunctivally below the lateral tarsus as a bolus allowing it to diffuse across the whole lid aided by pressure and massage if necessary. This tries to avoid a haematoma from the injection. It should be possible to do the procedure with the minimum bleeding and bruising especially if a radiofrequency, laser or other haemostatic and cutting instrument is used. If further anaesthesia is required it can always be given later under direct vision.
2. Place a traction suture in the middle of the lower tarsal plate and evert the lid over a Desmarres' retractor.
3. Cut through the conjunctiva with a blade 4 mm below the lower border of the tarsus. Cauterise the underlying lower lid retractors before cutting them (Fig 12.9). Other cutting and haemostatic instruments can be used as desired provided the necessary precautions are taken such as corneal protection using an appropriate contact lens with laser surgery.
4. Identify the lower lid fat by gently exploring the open space between the lower lid retractors and orbicularis muscle.
5. Place a traction suture in the flap of conjunctiva and lower lid retractors which can be pulled up to protect the cornea.
6. Remove the Desmarres' retractor and reinsert it to pull the orbicularis muscle forwards. This creates a better exposure of the fat and allows the preseptal space between the orbital septum and orbicularis muscle to be opened down to the orbital rim. It can be extended further to create a pocket over the suborbicularis oculi fat pat if desired. The fat can be excised and cauterised as required.
7. The attachment of the inferior orbital septum to the arcus marginalis can be opened if desired and the lower lid fat mobilised as with a skin/muscle flap blepharoplasty. Try to achieve complete haemostasis.
8. Remove the lower lid traction sutures and leave the posterior wound open to granulate or put one buried 6 or 7 '0' absorbable suture in the middle of the wound to gently approximate the conjunctival wound edges.
   Note: If the lid is lax it can be tightened at the lateral canthus with a suture or lateral canthal sling as previously described.

Complications

Visual loss. This can occur but since the posterior wound is effectively left open it is rare.

Lid retraction. This can occur if the wound is closed but should not do so if the wound is left open or only one suture is used to gently approximate the conjunctival edges.

Postoperative bleeding. This can occur from the open granulating wound but is usually easily controlled. Tell the patient in an emergency to use the palm of the hand to gently press on the eyelids and if the bleeding does not rapidly stop to pad the eye closed for a short period such as 6–12 hours.

BROW LIFT

The brow position is controlled by the frontalis muscle which elevates the brow, and the corrugator, procerus and orbital orbicularis muscles which all depress the brow. Their importance can be demonstrated by paralysing them with botulinum toxin which allows the frontalis muscle to act without its antagonists and causes a so-called 'chemical brow lift'. This can be a very desirable side effect of trying to eliminate the glabella frown lines with botulinum toxin but it is of course short-lived.

With age tissues stretch and the brow tends to drop with gravity. It can be raised with a variety of techniques, the simplest of which is the direct brow lift. This is effective but the scar is relatively unpredictable. It remains the procedure of choice for patients with 7th nerve palsy and paralysis of the frontalis muscle. Other techniques in which the scar is better camouflaged include the mid forehead, temporal and endoscopic lifts. The principles of these are given here but larger textbooks more specifically devoted to cosmetic surgery need to be consulted for further details. The so-called internal brow lift or brow stabilising suture is included as it is a relatively simple adjunct to a blepharoplasty which is useful for helping to support the brow and prevent it from drooping further when excess temporal eyelid tissue is excised.

The mid-forehead lift is particularly useful in men whose hairline may recede. It involves excising an elipse of skin and subcutaneous tissue in the line of the forehead furrows. A portion of the frontalis muscle is resected and the tissue closed in layers. The scar should blend with the forehead creases. It does not provide a very effective lift, although its efficiency can be improved with deep fixation sutures.

The temporal lift involves excising an elipse of skin and subcutaneous tissue down to the deep temporalis fascia behind the hairline and above the ear. The deep tissues can be undermined safely by staying on the deep temporalis fascia and not extending further forward than a line drawn from the tragus to a point 1 cm above the tail of the brow, which is the surface marking for the temporal branch of the facial nerve.

The endoscopic lift involves making a series of sagittal incisions about 2 cm behind the forehead hairline. The periosteum is elevated between these incisions down to the orbital rim where it is released under endoscopic control, taking care to preserve the supraorbital nerve and vessels. The corrugator and procerus muscles are excised. The periosteum is pulled upwards to elevate the brow and is fixed to the bone at a higher level with various devices.

DIRECT BROW LIFT (Fig 12.10)

Principle

An elipse of skin, orbicularis and frontalis muscle is excised at the upper border of the brow hairs. This resection elevates the brow but if there is a 7th nerve palsy the deep tissues are sutured to the periosteum for additional support. The resection can be carried out across the whole brow or any part of it e.g. temporally to elevate a temporal brow ptosis. The scar is unpredictable but it may be camouflaged by breaking up the line of the incision. The frontal nerve is at risk if

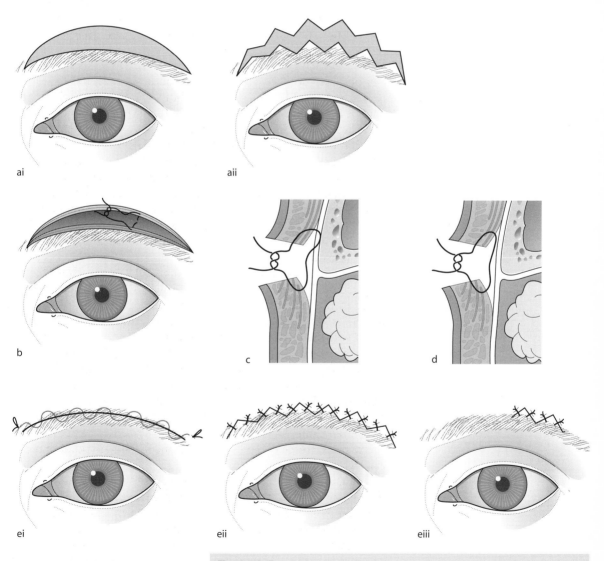

ai

aii

b

c

d

ei

eii

eiii

Figure 12.10

the incision and resection is not kept superficial in the region of the supraorbital notch.

Indications

Correction of a brow ptosis from any cause e.g. 7th nerve palsy, involutional changes, etc. The brow position should be assessed in all patients prior to a blepharoplasty.

Method

1. Mark the upper border of the eyebrow just in the hairline.
2. Estimate the extent of the required excision by pushing up the brow with the eyelids closed. Mark this on the skin (Fig 12.10ai).
   Note: For cosmetic purposes the scar may be better camouflaged if the incision is staggered as in Fig 12.10aii and/or is confined to a small area centred on the junction of the lateral third with the medial two-thirds of the brow (Fig 12.10eiii).
3. Inject local anaesthetic if not under general anaesthesia.
4. Excise skin, orbicularis and frontalis muscle down to the periosteum but try to identify and preserve the frontal nerve which passes under the supraorbital notch.
5. If there is a 7th nerve palsy, suture the deep fascia of the eyebrow to the periosteum with interrupted 4 '0' nonabsorbable sutures such as nylon or prolene (Fig 12.10b,c). If the frontalis muscle is active close the wound with long-acting absorbable sutures that do not pick up the periosteum (Fig 12.10d).
6. Close the deep layers of the wound with absorbable sutures and the skin with a continuous subcuticular pull out suture (Fig 12.10ei). If interrupted sutures are used as may be necessary with a staggered incision (Fig 12.10eii and 12.10eiii) they should be removed in 4 days or they may cause suture marks in the thick forehead skin.

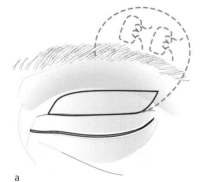

a

Complications

Visible scar. It may be possible to camouflage the scar by breaking it up with a staggered incision as described above.

Anaesthesia in the distribution of the frontal nerve if it is accidentally cut.

INTERNAL BROW LIFT (BROW STABILISING SUTURE) (Fig 12.11)

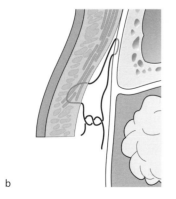

b

Figure 12.11

Principle

The brow is supported by deep nonabsorbable sutures placed in the periosteum above the orbital rim which is exposed as part of an upper lid blepharoplasty procedure (Fig 12.11a,b).

Indications

Mild brow ptosis especially temporally when the patient does not want a scar or need a more major procedure. The suture is useful in helping to support the brow and prevent any increase in temporal brow ptosis which may appear to occur when temporal 'hoods' are excised (Fig 12.11a).

Method

Stages 1–9 as for upper lid blepharoplasty

10. Expose the periosteum over the frontal bone by undermining the brow fat pad from the orbital septum and periosteum over the orbital rim.

    Note: Do not undermine the brow fat pad from the orbicularis muscle or excise any fat until you have assessed the effect of the brow stabilising sutures as they will alter the appearance of the excess brow fat.

11. Retract the upper lid skin and brow with a Desmarres', malleable or other retractor. Place a permanent suture e.g. 4 '0' prolene directly into the frontal periosteum. If it is not possible to get adequate exposure to do this via the blepharoplasty incision, the needle can be introduced through the forehead skin, through all the tissues and passed into the periosteum to get as good a bit as possible. The needle is then brought out through the blepharoplasty incision and the other end of the suture is similarly pulled out through the same incision by pulling the suture through the tissues with a squint hook, leaving the bite through the periosteum.

12. Hold the 4 '0' prolene needle in a general purpose needle holder. Find the area of the brow that you want to lift by pushing up the deep tissues of the brow with the back of the needle. Take a good bite of the tissues at this point and try the elevating effect of tightening the suture (Fig 12.11b). If this is not satisfactory replace the suture.

13. Do the same to the other side and add more sutures as desired to both sides. Then tighten and tie the least effective sutures and do the same for the other sutures to try and get as symmetrical a result as possible.

14. Complete the upper lid blepharoplasty stages 10–16.

    Note: It is rarely necessary to debulk the brow fat pad if brow stabilising sutures have been used as they lift up and support the brow fat pad.

Complications

Pain over the periosteal suture bites. Dimpling of the tissues if the sutures are placed too superficially. Both these complications tend to resolve with time although the wound can be opened and sutures removed if desired.

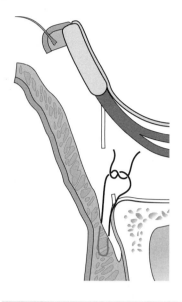

Figure 12.12

CHEEK LIFT

PRE SOOF LIFT (Fig 12.12)

Principle

The cheek tissues are supported and lifted by suturing the suborbicularis tissue over the suborbicularis fat pad to the periosteum of the orbital rim (Fig 12.12).

Indications

A mild degree of cheek ptosis. A supramalar sulcus or tear trough deformity when the patient has little or no lower lid fat which can be released.

Method

Stages 1–8 as for skin/muscle lower lid blepharoplasty.

9. Free the orbicularis muscle from the orbital rim and create a space under the orbicularis muscle and over the suborbicularis fat pad.
10. Use forceps to hold the suborbicularis fascial tissue in various places and assess the effect of pulling the cheek up to the orbital rim.
11. When satisfied place a suture such as 4 '0' prolene through the suborbicularis fascial tissue in the position of the forceps, then through the orbital rim periosteum and tie it. If it is not satisfactory replace it.
12. Repeat this three or four times around the inferior orbital rim on both sides.
13. Complete the skin/muscle blepharoplasty stages 10–12.

Complications

Prolonged lower lid oedema. Dimpling of the skin. Both of these usually resolve with time but may take months to do so.

SOOF LIFT (Fig 12.13)

Principle

The cheek tissues are lifted by separating the cheek periosteum from the underlying bone, freeing it at its lower end to allow it to be pulled superiorly and resuturing it to the periosteum of the orbital rim (Fig 12.13). Care must be taken to preserve the infraorbital nerve. It is often combined with a lower lid hard palate mucosal graft and lateral canthal surgery to elevate the lower lid as well as the cheek.

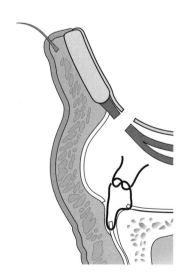

Figure 12.13

Indications

Marked cheek ptosis whether involutional or due to 7th nerve palsy. Lid retraction which can be corrected by pushing the cheek up with a finger and is not correctable by lateral canthal surgery alone in whom a skin graft is cosmetically undesirable.

Method

Stages 1–6 as for a skin/muscle blepharoplasty or stages 1–3 as for a lateral canthal approach to the orbital floor (swinging eyelid flap) if it is proposed to carry out lateral canthal surgery and insert a hard palate mucosal graft.

7. Expose the periosteum and cut through it along the orbital rim just anterior to the arcus marginalis.
8. Identify the position of the infra orbital nerve foramen and make a short vertical cut through the periosteum to expose the nerve and preserve it. Use periosteal elevators to lift the periosteum on either side of the nerve and continue raising it as far as the superior gingival sulcus.
9. If pulling up the periosteum does not allow the cheek to be elevated satisfactorily cut through the attached lower edge of the periosteum with an angled beaver blade or scleral pocket knife.
10. When the cheek can be elevated adequately pull it up and fix it by suturing the malar periosteum to the arcus marginalis with a series of buried nonabsorbable sutures such as 4 '0' prolene (Fig. 12.13).

Complete the surgery as appropriate e.g. stages 7–12 for lower lid skin/muscle blepharoplasty, stages 8–9 for lateral canthal approach to orbital floor with or without a hard palate mucosal graft as for lower lid retractor lengthening (p 200); and with lateral canthal surgery as per chapter on ectropion.

Complications

Hypo-aesthesia or anaesthesia in the distribution of the infraorbital nerve.

Index